I0037363

Revolutionizing Cancer Treatment Strategies

Revolutionizing Cancer Treatment Strategies

Maria .M

Noble Publishing

CONTENTS ▌

INDEX

6.3 Current research and developments in nanomedicine

Chapter 7: Artificial Intelligence in Oncology
7.1 The role of artificial intelligence in cancer diagnosis and treatment
7.2 Machine learning algorithms for predicting treatment outcomes
7.3 Examples of AI applications in cancer research and treatment

Chapter 8: Patient-Centered Approaches
8.1 Importance of considering the patient's perspective in cancer treatment
8.2 Integrating holistic care and supportive therapies
8.3 Highlighting successful patient-centered approaches

Chapter 9: Future Prospects and Challenges
9.1 Exploration of emerging trends in cancer research and treatment
9.2 Anticipated challenges and ethical considerations
9.3 Call to action for continued innovation in cancer treatment strategies

Chapter 1

Introduction

Malignant growth, a considerable enemy that has tormented mankind over now is the ideal time, keeps on being a significant worldwide wellbeing challenge in the 21st 100 years. Notwithstanding significant advancement in how we might interpret the basic sub-atomic systems and the improvement of different therapy modalities, the intricacy and flexibility of malignant growth cells have frustrated numerous regular remedial methodologies. The mission to upset disease treatment procedures has turned into an objective, driven by the pressing need to upgrade viability, limit secondary effects, and at last work on understanding results.

The scene of disease treatment has gone through huge changes throughout the long term. From the beginning of a medical procedure as the essential mediation to the coming of chemotherapy and radiation treatment, the field has seen exceptional progressions. In any case, these conventional methodologies have limits, frequently making blow-back sound tissues and prompting crippling secondary effects. The rise of designated treatments denoted a change in perspective, offering a more exact and customized approach by straightforwardly disrupting explicit sub-atomic pathways embroiled in malignant growth movement. By and by, challenges continue, including the improvement of obstruction and the heterogeneity of malignant growth cells inside a solitary cancer.

As of late, the combination of different logical disciplines has brought about novel and promising roads in the fight against malignant growth. The incorporation of genomics, immunology, man-made consciousness, and nanotechnology has opened new wildernesses, permitting scientists and clinicians to investigate creative treatment modalities. This multi-layered approach means to take advantage of the novel qualities of malignant growth cells while limiting damage to ordinary tissues, introducing another period of accuracy medication in oncology.

Genomic experiences play had a significant impact in unwinding the intricacies of disease. The appearance of high-throughput sequencing advances has empowered the exhaustive profiling of malignant growth genomes, working with the ID of key hereditary adjustments driving tumorigenesis. Accuracy oncology, a methodology that tailors treatment in view of the hereditary cosmetics of a singular's growth, has picked up speed. Atomically designated treatments, like tyrosine kinase inhibitors and resistant designated spot inhibitors, represent the progress of this methodology in unambiguous malignant growth subtypes. The continuous endeavors to interpret the genomic scene of different tumors hold the commitment of distinguishing novel helpful targets and refining treatment techniques further.

Immunotherapy, when considered a specialty approach, has arisen as a unique advantage in malignant growth treatment. Outfitting the body's safe framework to perceive and kill disease cells, immunotherapy has exhibited phenomenal outcome in specific malignancies. Designated spot inhibitors, fanciful antigen receptor (Vehicle) Lymphocyte treatment, and disease antibodies address the different armory of immunotherapeutic intercessions. The capacity to prompt solid reactions and, at times, accomplish long haul reduction has energized hopefulness about the groundbreaking capability of immunotherapy across a range of tumors.

The multifaceted interchange among disease and the resistant framework has prodded continuous examination to disentangle the systems of invulnerable avoidance utilized by cancers. Mix treatments, consolidating immunomodulatory specialists with customary therapies or different immunotherapies, are being investigated to improve the general enemy of malignant growth insusceptible reaction. The powerful idea of the invulnerable growth cooperation presents the two difficulties and open doors, requiring a nuanced understanding to upgrade helpful results.

Computerized reasoning (artificial intelligence) has penetrated different aspects of malignant growth research and clinical work on, offering exceptional computational power and scientific capacities. AI calculations examine immense datasets, including genomic profiles, clinical imaging, and clinical records, to distinguish examples and connections that might evade human perception. Man-made intelligence driven prescient models help in risk delineation, early discovery, and treatment arranging. Besides, the reconciliation of artificial intelligence in drug revelation facilitates the distinguishing proof of novel mixtures and potential medication blends, speeding up the improvement of designated treatments.

The coming of nanotechnology has given an exceptional stage to the designated conveyance of restorative specialists to disease cells. Nanoparticles, designed to convey medications or imaging specialists, can take advantage of the improved penetrability and maintenance impact of growth vasculature, specifically collecting in the growth microenvironment. This designated approach limits openness to sound tissues and improves the helpful record of hostile to malignant growth specialists. Also, nanotechnology works with the advancement of theranostic stages, joining remedial and analytic functionalities to screen treatment reaction continuously.

The transformation in malignant growth treatment stretches out past the research facility and center to the domain of patient consideration and survivorship. Patient-driven approaches focus on personal satisfaction, mental prosperity, and long haul results. Strong consideration intercessions, going from integrative treatments to psychosocial support, plan to alleviate the physical and profound weights of disease treatment. Survivorship programs address the exceptional necessities of people post-treatment, zeroing in on reconnaissance, wellbeing support, and the avoidance of long haul sequelae.

The quest for progressive disease treatment methodologies requires cooperative endeavors across disciplines and worldwide limits. Research consortia, like The Disease Genome Chart book (TCGA) and the Worldwide Malignant growth Genome Consortium (ICGC), embody worldwide drives to gather and share genomic information, cultivating a cooperative climate for logical disclosure. Open-access stages and information sharing drives speed up the interpretation of examination discoveries into clinical applications, expanding the effect on tolerant consideration.

While the scene of disease therapy is advancing quickly, moves continue on the way to altering malignant growth care. The intrinsic heterogeneity of malignant growth, both between and inside individual cancers, represents an impressive snag. Cancer advancement, clonal elements, and the rise of treatment safe subpopulations highlight the requirement for dynamic and versatile therapy systems. Additionally, the moral contemplations encompassing genomic information protection, the fair dispersion of imaginative treatments, and the possible cultural ramifications of trend setting innovations require cautious route.

The monetary ramifications of carrying out clever disease medicines additionally warrant thought. The expense of creating and conveying state of the art treatments, combined with the monetary weight of malignant growth care, brings up issues about availability and moderateness. Finding some kind of harmony among development and inclusivity is fundamental to guarantee that forward leaps in malignant growth treatment benefit a wide and various populace.

As we stand at the edge of another period in malignant growth treatment, the basic to address these difficulties is matched exclusively by the phenomenal open doors that lie ahead. The union of genomics, immunology, man-made consciousness, and nanotechnology has synergistically impelled the field forward, offering a diverse way to deal with battle malignant growth. The continuous investigation of the growth microenvironment, the unwinding of insusceptible growth connections, and the recognizable proof of novel restorative targets keep on extending how we might interpret disease science.

In the excursion to change disease treatment procedures, the job of interdisciplinary cooperation couldn't possibly be more significant. Clinicians, researchers, designers, and ethicists merge in an aggregate work to make an interpretation of logical revelations into unmistakable advantages for patients. The joining of different viewpoints guarantees a complete and comprehensive way to deal with malignant growth care, tending to the natural complexities of the infection as well as the more extensive parts of patient prosperity and cultural effect.

All in all, the scene of disease treatment is going through a significant change, powered by progressions in genomics, immunology, computerized reasoning, and nanotechnology. The quest for accuracy medication, immunotherapy, and designated mediations proclaims another time wherein the intricacies of disease are met with imaginative and customized arrangements. As we explore the difficulties and open doors on this excursion, a definitive objective remaining parts undaunted: to change malignant growth treatment procedures and usher in a time where the finding isn't inseparable from despair, yet rather a source of inspiration for a more successful, caring, and available way to deal with vanquishing this imposing enemy.

1.1 Overview of the current state of cancer treatment

Malignant growth, an inescapable and diverse sickness, keeps on testing the worldwide medical services scene, requiring a dynamic and developing way to deal with therapy. The present status of disease therapy mirrors a different cluster of modalities, from customary mediations like a medical procedure, chemotherapy, and radiation treatment to later headways in accuracy medication, immunotherapy, and designated treatments. Understanding the qualities and restrictions of these methodologies is pivotal in exploring the complicated landscape of malignant growth care.

Medical procedure, a foundation of disease therapy for quite a long time, stays an essential methodology for limited cancers. The objective of careful mediation is to extract the malignant tissue while safeguarding encompassing sound designs. Propels in careful methods, including negligibly obtrusive strategies and automated helped a medical procedure, have added to diminished recuperation times and worked on post-operative results. In any case, the adequacy of medical procedure is dependent upon elements like growth area, size, and the shortfall of metastasis.

Chemotherapy, a sturdy in disease therapy, includes the organization of cytotoxic medications to obliterate or repress the development of quickly separating malignant growth cells. While chemotherapy has shown adequacy in different malignancies, its vague nature can prompt blow-back to sound cells, bringing about crippling secondary effects. The journey for additional designated and less harmful treatments brought about the time of designated treatments.

Designated treatments address a change in perspective in disease treatment, expecting to slow down unambiguous sub-atomic pathways engaged with cancer development and movement. Tyrosine kinase inhibitors, for instance, disturb flagging pathways ensnared in disease cell multiplication, while chemical receptor blockers restrain the development advancing impacts of chemicals in chemical touchy malignant growths. Designated treatments offer a more exact methodology than customary chemotherapy, with the potential for upgraded viability and diminished poisonousness. Be that as it may, difficulties, for example, the improvement of opposition and the heterogeneity of malignant growth cells inside a cancer present continuous obstacles.

Radiation treatment utilizes ionizing radiation to harm the DNA of malignant growth cells, restraining their capacity to multiply. It is a significant part of malignant growth treatment, frequently utilized related to a medical procedure or as an independent treatment. Mechanical headways, for example, power balanced radiation treatment (IMRT) and proton treatment, empower more exact focusing of growths while saving neighboring sound tissues. Regardless of these upgrades, radiation treatment can in any case prompt secondary effects, stressing the requirement for proceeded with refinement in conveyance methods.

Accuracy medication, established in the comprehension of the sub-atomic and hereditary premise of disease, addresses a momentous way to deal with treatment. Genomic profiling of growths takes into consideration the ID of explicit hereditary adjustments driving disease movement. This information empowers the determination of designated treatments custom fitted to the special qualities of a singular's disease. Microscopically designated treatments, including epidermal development factor receptor (EGFR) inhibitors and BRAF inhibitors, epitomize the progress of accuracy medication in specific disease subtypes. The continuous investigation of the genomic scene holds the commitment of revealing new remedial targets and refining treatment procedures further.

Immunotherapy, a progressive road in disease therapy, bridles the body's safe framework to perceive and take out malignant growth cells. Designated spot inhibitors, like customized cell demise protein 1 (PD-1) and cytotoxic T-lymphocyte-related protein 4 (CTLA-4) inhibitors, release the resistant framework's capacity to mount an enemy of disease reaction. Illusory antigen receptor (Vehicle) Lymphocyte treatment includes designing a patient's own Immune system microorganisms to target explicit disease antigens.

Immunotherapy has shown noteworthy outcome in specific malignancies, with tough reactions and, now and again, long haul abatement. Be that as it may, not all patients answer, and insusceptible related unfriendly occasions highlight the requirement for a nuanced comprehension of the complicated interaction among disease and the invulnerable framework.

Man-made reasoning (man-made intelligence) has arisen as a groundbreaking power in disease research and clinical practice. AI calculations investigate tremendous datasets, including genomic profiles, clinical imaging, and clinical records, to recognize examples and connections. Artificial intelligence driven prescient models help in risk definition, early discovery, and treatment arranging. The joining of computer based intelligence in drug revelation speeds up the distinguishing proof of novel mixtures and potential medication blends, speeding up the advancement of designated treatments. The collaboration among simulated intelligence and conventional examination systems holds the possibility to open new bits of knowledge and push the field forward.

Nanotechnology, with its ability for exact control at the nanoscale, offers creative arrangements in malignant growth treatment. Nanoparticles, designed to convey restorative specialists, can take advantage of the remarkable qualities of the growth microenvironment for designated drug conveyance. This approach limits openness to sound tissues, upgrading the remedial record of hostile to disease specialists. In addition, nanotechnology works with the improvement of theranostic stages, consolidating helpful and symptomatic functionalities to screen treatment reaction continuously. The mix of nanotechnology into disease therapeutics proclaims another period of accuracy and viability.

The scene of disease therapy stretches out past the domain of clinical mediations to envelop strong consideration and survivorship. Steady consideration mediations, going from torment the executives to psychosocial support, mean to improve the general prosperity of patients going through disease treatment. Palliative consideration, zeroed in on side effect alleviation and personal satisfaction, is a fundamental part of the extensive consideration continuum. Survivorship programs address the interesting requirements of people post-treatment, stressing reconnaissance, wellbeing upkeep, and the administration of treatment-related sequelae.

The present status of malignant growth treatment is portrayed by a powerful interaction between customary modalities and state of the art developments. Multidisciplinary coordinated effort, including oncologists, specialists, radiologists, pathologists, and analysts, is fundamental for fitting treatment plans to individual patients. Growth sheets, where specialists from different disciplines gather to talk about complex cases, represent the cooperative methodology that supports present day disease care. Furthermore, patient association in dynamic cycles and the reconciliation of patient-detailed results add to a more understanding driven worldview.

Clinical preliminaries, the foundation of translational exploration, assume an essential part in propelling disease treatment. Investigational medications and treatments go through thorough assessment in clinical preliminaries to survey security, viability, and possible secondary effects. The ever-evolving refinement of treatment conventions and the approval of novel helpful methodologies depend on the support of patients in clinical preliminaries. The joining of certifiable proof and creative preliminary plans further upgrades the effectiveness and generalizability of preliminary results.

Regardless of the headway made in disease treatment, imposing difficulties persevere. The heterogeneity of disease, both at the sub-atomic and cell levels, requires a nuanced comprehension of growth science. Cancer advancement, clonal elements, and the rise of treatment safe subpopulations highlight the requirement for dynamic and versatile therapy methodologies. The recognizable proof of solid biomarkers for treatment reaction and opposition stays a complicated undertaking, requiring progressing research endeavors.

The monetary ramifications of malignant growth treatment additionally warrant thought. The expense of creating and conveying state of the art treatments, combined with the financial weight of disease care, brings up issues about availability and moderateness. Abberations in admittance to creative medicines, both inside and across nations, feature the requirement for impartial conveyance and asset designation. Finding some kind of harmony among development and inclusivity is fundamental to guarantee that advances in malignant growth treatment benefit a wide and different populace.

Moral contemplations pose a potential threat in the scene of malignant growth treatment, especially with the coming of accuracy medication and genomic profiling. Inquiries of information security, assent, and the potential for unseen side-effects require watchful oversight and moral structures. Adjusting the basic for logical headway with moral standards guarantees that advancement in disease treatment lines up with the more extensive objectives of working on persistent results and cultural prosperity.

All in all, the present status of disease treatment mirrors a unique exchange among custom and development. From revered modalities, for example, medical procedure and chemotherapy to state of the art approaches like accuracy medication, immunotherapy, and nanotechnology, the stockpile against malignant growth keeps on extending. Multidisciplinary cooperation, patient-focused care, and progressing research endeavors drive the development of disease treatment systems. As we explore the intricacies of malignant growth, the basic is clear: to constantly refine and change our methodology, taking a stab at a future where the conclusion of disease is met with viable, designated, and caring arrangements that work on the existences of people and networks around the world.

1.2 Statistics on cancer prevalence and the impact on global health

Disease, a perplexing and different gathering of illnesses portrayed by uncontrolled cell development, addresses a huge worldwide wellbeing challenge. The commonness of disease has been consistently ascending, with significant ramifications for people, networks, and medical services frameworks around the world. A far reaching assessment of the measurements on disease commonness gives bits of knowledge into the size of the issue, the circulation of malignant growth types, and the financial effect on worldwide wellbeing.

The sheer size of disease's effect becomes evident while thinking about its commonness on a worldwide scale. As per the World Wellbeing Association (WHO), disease is one of the main sources of dreariness and mortality around the world, representing an expected 9.6 million passings in 2018. The occurrence of new disease cases is likewise on the ascent, with roughly 18.1 million new cases analyzed in 2018. These figures highlight the critical requirement for an organized and complete reaction to address the developing weight of disease.

The dissemination of malignant growth types shifts across locales, mirroring a complicated transaction of hereditary, ecological, and way of life factors. Cellular breakdown in the lungs reliably positions as the most widely recognized malignant growth worldwide, with a significant piece of cases credited to tobacco smoking. Bosom disease follows intently, especially among ladies, while colorectal, stomach, and liver tumors likewise contribute fundamentally to the worldwide malignant growth trouble. Local varieties in disease commonness feature the significance of fitting anticipation, early identification, and treatment techniques to the particular epidemiological qualities of every populace.

Past the mathematical information, the effect of disease reaches out past individual wellbeing results to cultural and financial aspects. The financial weight of malignant growth includes direct clinical expenses, for example, indicative and treatment costs, as well as aberrant costs connected with efficiency misfortune and untimely mortality. The monetary stress on medical care frameworks and people is significant, with malignant growth frequently requiring delayed and asset concentrated therapy regimens.

Notwithstanding financial outcomes, the psychosocial effect of malignant growth resonates through networks and families. A malignant growth finding can involve profound trouble, disturbances to day to day existence, and difficulties in keeping up with social connections. The far reaching influences stretch out to guardians, who bear a huge weight in offering help and exploring the intricacies of disease care. Addressing the psychosocial parts of disease is necessary to a comprehensive methodology that thinks about the actual prosperity of people as well as their psychological and profound wellbeing.

Age is a basic consider malignant growth pervasiveness, with the gamble of creating disease expanding fundamentally with propelling age. As populaces age internationally, the weight of malignant growth is supposed to correspondingly rise. This segment shift presents novel difficulties, as more seasoned people might confront extra intricacies in malignant growth the executives, including comorbidities, feebleness, and adjusted drug digestion. Fitting malignant growth care to the particular necessities of more seasoned grown-ups is fundamental for improving treatment results and guaranteeing an honorable personal satisfaction.

Topographical variations in disease pervasiveness further highlight the requirement for designated mediations and asset portion. Low-and center pay nations bear a lopsided weight of malignant growth, with higher death rates and less assets for counteraction, early recognition, and treatment. Restricted admittance to medical services foundation, including disease screening and symptomatic offices, worsens the difficulties looked by these districts. Overcoming any issues in malignant growth care between big time salary and low-pay nations requires a coordinated work to address foundational obstructions and advance worldwide value in medical services.

Preventive estimates assume a significant part in relieving the effect of malignant growth on worldwide wellbeing. Way of life factors, for example, tobacco use, unfortunate eating regimens, actual idleness, and openness to natural cancer-causing agents contribute fundamentally to disease risk. Endeavors to lessen tobacco utilization, advance solid dietary propensities, and establish conditions that help actual work are vital parts of malignant growth avoidance methodologies. Inoculation against irresistible specialists connected to explicit tumors, for example, human papillomavirus (HPV) and hepatitis B infection (HBV), further epitomizes the preventive methodology.

Early location of malignant growth is significant for further developing treatment results and diminishing mortality. Evaluating programs for specific malignant growths, like bosom, cervical, and colorectal diseases, intend to recognize precancerous sores or beginning phase cancers when mediations are best. Notwithstanding, the execution of screening programs faces difficulties connected with access, adherence, and the accessibility of medical care foundation. Training and mindfulness crusades assume an imperative part in advancing the significance of early location and empowering people to take part in screening drives.

Progressions in demonstrative advancements, including imaging modalities and atomic profiling, have upgraded the accuracy and effectiveness of malignant growth conclusion. The incorporation of genomics and biomarker examination takes into consideration more precise growth characterization, directing therapy choices in light of the extraordinary hereditary profile of every disease. Sub-atomic diagnostics, for example, fluid biopsy methods, hold guarantee for painless malignant growth recognition and checking, reforming the scene of early disease conclusion.

Therapy modalities for disease incorporate a different exhibit of choices, going from a medical procedure and chemotherapy to radiation treatment, immunotherapy, and designated treatments. The determination of therapy relies upon elements, for example, disease type, stage, and individual patient attributes. Careful intercessions plan to eliminate limited growths, frequently supplemented by adjuvant treatments to target remaining disease cells. Chemotherapy, while related with incidental effects, stays a foundation of malignant growth treatment, especially for fundamental sicknesses.

The coming of designated treatments denotes a groundbreaking period in malignant growth treatment. These treatments explicitly target sub-atomic pathways engaged with disease development and movement, offering a more exact and custom fitted methodology than conventional chemotherapy. Tyrosine kinase inhibitors, chemical receptor blockers, and resistant designated spot inhibitors represent the progress of designated treatments in specific disease subtypes. The continuous ID of novel helpful focuses through genomic research keeps on growing the collection of designated intercessions.

Immunotherapy addresses a change in perspective in malignant growth therapy by saddling the body's safe framework to perceive and take out disease cells. Designated spot inhibitors, Vehicle White blood cell treatment, and disease immunizations epitomize the assorted range of immunotherapeutic methodologies. The outcome of immunotherapy in accomplishing tough reactions and, at times, long haul reduction highlights its expected across a scope of malignancies. The unique idea of the invulnerable cancer connection, be that as it may, presents difficulties connected with reaction changeability and safe related antagonistic occasions.

Radiation treatment, using ionizing radiation to target and obliterate disease cells, stays a critical part of malignant growth therapy. Innovative headways, including picture directed radiation treatment (IGRT) and proton treatment, improve the accuracy of radiation conveyance while limiting harm to encompassing sound tissues. The coordination of radiation treatment with other therapy modalities, like a medical procedure and chemotherapy, streamlines restorative results in a multidisciplinary approach.

The coming of computerized reasoning (simulated intelligence) has catalyzed a transformation in disease examination, conclusion, and treatment. AI calculations examine immense datasets, including genomic profiles, clinical imaging, and clinical records, to distinguish examples and connections. Artificial intelligence driven prescient models help in risk separation, early recognition, and treatment arranging. The coordination of artificial intelligence in drug disclosure facilitates the distinguishing proof of novel mixtures and potential medication blends, speeding up the advancement of designated treatments. The cooperative energy among man-made intelligence and customary examination strategies holds the possibility to open new bits of knowledge and drive the field forward.

Nanotechnology offers imaginative arrangements in malignant growth treatment by utilizing the remarkable properties of materials at the nanoscale. Nanoparticles, designed to convey helpful specialists, can specifically target malignant growth cells while limiting openness to solid tissues. This designated drug conveyance approach improves the restorative list of hostile to malignant growth specialists and lessens fundamental incidental effects. The mix of nanotechnology into malignant growth therapeutics additionally works with the improvement of theranostic stages, joining helpful and indicative functionalities for continuous treatment observing.

1.3 Introduction to the need for revolutionary treatment strategies

In the domain of medical care, the never-ending quest for imaginative and progressive therapy procedures remains as a basic reaction to the consistently developing scene of sicknesses and clinical difficulties. As social orders progress and experience novel wellbeing dangers, the traditional strategies for determination and treatment frequently get themselves lacking in tending to the complexities of arising conditions. This requires a change in perspective in our methodology towards medical care, convincing us to investigate and embrace progressive therapy systems that can rethink the limits of clinical conceivable outcomes.

The direness for progressive therapy methodologies is highlighted by the limits of conventional clinical mediations notwithstanding intricate and dynamic medical problems. Illnesses, both irresistible and non-transferable, keep on advancing, introducing extraordinary difficulties to the medical services environment. Besides, the rising interconnectedness of the worldwide populace and the simplicity of movement add to the quick spread of infections, requesting a quick and versatile reaction from the clinical local area.

By and large, the improvement of treatment methodologies has been a progressive and iterative cycle, set apart by steady headways in figuring out sicknesses and refining restorative methodologies. Nonetheless, the contemporary medical care scene requests a takeoff from this incrementalism, requiring a more progressive position to face the diverse difficulties that have arisen as of late.

One of the main thrusts behind the requirement for progressive treatment techniques is the ascent of antimicrobial opposition (AMR). Overreliance on anti-microbials and other antimicrobial specialists has prompted the advancement of medication safe kinds of microscopic organisms and different microorganisms, de-livering once-successful medicines insufficient. This approaching danger imperils the groundwork of current medication, as standard operations, from medical procedures to chemotherapy, become progressively unsafe because of the potential for untreatable diseases.

The ongoing direction of AMR proposes a future where normal diseases may indeed become hazardous, suggestive of a pre-anti-infection period. To deflect such an emergency, progressive treatment methodologies are basic, including the improve-ment of new antimicrobial specialists as well as a principal reconsideration of how we approach contamination counteraction, conclusion, and treatment.

Past irresistible infections, the rising predominance of constant circumstances like cardiovascular illnesses, diabetes, and malignant growth adds one more layer of intricacy to the medical services challenge. Customary medicines for these afflictions frequently center around side effect the executives as opposed to tending to the main drivers. A progressive methodology includes a shift towards accuracy medication, fitting medicines in light of individual hereditary cosmetics, way of life, and natural elements. This customized approach holds the commitment of additional compelling and designated mediations, possibly changing the scene of constant illness the board.

Notwithstanding the biomedical perspectives, the requirement for progressive therapy techniques is highlighted by the more extensive financial variables impacting medical services. Wellbeing variations persevere worldwide, with minimized networks confronting inconsistent admittance to medical services assets. Progressive method-ologies should zero in on clinical forward leaps as well as address the foundational imbalances that add to wellbeing disparities.

Mechanical headways assume a crucial part in driving the requirement for pro-gressive treatment systems. The coming of computerized reasoning (simulated in-telligence), AI, and enormous information examination has introduced another time of medical services, offering exceptional open doors for finding, therapy enhance-ment, and prescient demonstrating. Coordinating these advances into clinical practice requires a change in perspective in medical care conveyance, requiring changes in training, foundation, and administrative systems.

Besides, the rising intricacy of illnesses requests interdisciplinary cooperation, separating the conventional storehouses that have described clinical examination and practice. Progressive treatment systems frequently arise at the convergence of different logical disciplines, requiring an all encompassing and cooperative way to deal with innovative work.

Tending to the psychological wellness emergency addresses one more element of the call for progressive treatment methodologies. Psychological well-being conditions have arrived at pestilence extents, exacerbated by cultural tensions, financial vulnerabilities, and the shame encompassing dysfunctional behavior. The customary model of mental medical care, which frequently depends vigorously on drug mediations and psychotherapy, misses the mark in giving extensive and open arrangements.

A progressive way to deal with psychological well-being includes destigmatizing dysfunctional behaviors, coordinating emotional well-being into essential consideration, and utilizing mechanical arrangements, for example, telemedicine and computerized therapeutics. By embracing an all encompassing and patient-focused model, mental medical services can move past side effect the executives to advance long haul prosperity and versatility.

In addition, the natural difficulties of the 21st hundred years, including environmental change and ecological corruption, have significant ramifications for human wellbeing. The rising predominance of vector-borne illnesses, respiratory afflictions, and other medical problems connected to natural variables requires imaginative therapy procedures that recognize the reliance of human wellbeing and the climate.

All in all, the basic for progressive treatment procedures emerges from the multi-layered difficulties standing up to the contemporary medical care scene. From antimicrobial protection from persistent illnesses, wellbeing differences, mechanical interruptions, and natural dangers, the requirement for groundbreaking ways to deal with analysis, avoidance, and treatment is apparent. An extensive and interdisciplinary reaction, enveloping biomedical development, mechanical coordination, and fundamental changes, is vital for introduce another time of medical care that can successfully address the intricacies of 21st-century wellbeing challenges. Just through such a purposeful exertion could we at any point desire to guarantee the wellbeing and prosperity of current and people in the future.

In the steadily developing scene of medical services, the mission for progressive therapy procedures has turned into a vital pursuit, driven by the goals of tending to the intricacies of present day wellbeing challenges. The customary standards of clinical mediation are much of the time tracked down needing despite arising infections, advancing microbes, and the multifaceted exchange of hereditary, natural, and way of life factors. Thusly, the requirement for progressive treatment methodologies isn't simply a simple yearning yet a basic reaction to the dynamic and diverse nature of contemporary wellbeing concerns.

At the very front of the direness for progressive treatment systems is the heightening danger of antimicrobial opposition (AMR). The abuse and abuse of anti-toxins and other antimicrobial specialists have prompted the development of medication safe kinds of microbes and different microorganisms. This peculiarity imperils the actual groundwork of current medication, as normal operations, from medical procedures to chemotherapy, become progressively risky because of the potential for untreatable diseases.

Antimicrobial obstruction, whenever left uncontrolled, takes steps to dive us into a post-anti-infection period where once-treatable diseases can go lethal. The weightiness of this present circumstance requires a basic change in our way to deal with irresistible illnesses.

Progressive treatment procedures should go past the improvement of new antimicrobial specialists; they should envelop an all encompassing reconsideration of how we forestall, analyze, and treat contaminations. This remembers advancements for disease control rehearses, fast diagnostics, and elective treatment modalities.

The ascent of antimicrobial opposition highlights the interconnectedness of worldwide wellbeing and the requirement for cooperative endeavors on a global scale. The advancement of new anti-infection agents alone is deficient; facilitated activities to control and upgrade antimicrobial use, further develop reconnaissance frameworks, and improve worldwide readiness are vital parts of a thorough methodology against AMR.

Past irresistible illnesses, the commonness of persistent circumstances further underlines the need for progressive treatment procedures. A critical part of the worldwide infection trouble involves non-transmittable sicknesses like cardiovascular illnesses, diabetes, and malignant growth. Regular medicines for these circumstances frequently center around overseeing side effects instead of tending to the basic causes.

A change in perspective is expected to move from a responsive to a proactive methodology in medical services. This shift includes embracing accuracy medication — a progressive idea that tailors medicines in light of a person's hereditary cosmetics, way of life, and ecological elements. Accuracy medication holds the commitment of additional successful and designated intercessions, possibly changing the scene of ongoing sickness the executives.

The execution of accuracy medication, nonetheless, delivers its own arrangement of difficulties. It requires a reconfiguration of medical care frameworks to oblige the intricacies of individualized therapies. This remembers headways for hereditary testing, information examination, and the reconciliation of innovation to help customized medical care conveyance. Moreover, tending to moral contemplations, for example, protection concerns and impartial admittance to these high level medicines is fundamental in guaranteeing the capable and boundless reception of accuracy medication.

The financial components of medical care highlight the requirement for progressive therapy procedures that address foundational imbalances. Wellbeing inconsistencies continue all around the world, with minimized networks confronting hindrances to access and quality medical services. A far reaching way to deal with medical care change should incorporate measures to lessen these differences, guaranteeing that inventive therapies are open to all sections of the populace.

Mechanical headways assume a crucial part in driving the requirement for progressive treatment systems. The coming of man-made reasoning (computer based intelligence), AI, and huge information examination has introduced another time of medical care prospects.

These advances offer exceptional open doors for determination, treatment enhancement, and prescient demonstrating.

Man-made reasoning, specifically, can possibly reform clinical diagnostics. AI calculations can examine tremendous datasets, distinguishing examples and inconsistencies that might evade human discernment. This ability improves the exactness and effectiveness of symptomatic cycles, prompting prior and more exact distinguishing proof of sicknesses.

The incorporation of innovation into medical services, in any case, requires an extensive and versatile system. This includes defeating difficulties connected with information security, interoperability of frameworks, and the moral utilization of man-made consciousness in clinical direction. Administrative bodies assume a urgent part in laying out rules that offset development with patient wellbeing and moral contemplations.

Moreover, the rising intricacy of illnesses requests interdisciplinary coordinated effort, separating the customary storehouses that have portrayed clinical examination and practice. Progressive treatment techniques frequently arise at the convergence of different logical disciplines, requiring a comprehensive and cooperative way to deal with innovative work. Interdisciplinary groups containing specialists in medication, science, designing, and information science can encourage advancement by offering assorted points of view that would be useful.

As well as tending to explicit illnesses, progressive treatment methodologies ought to likewise include a more extensive point of view on medical care conveyance. This incorporates rethinking the patient experience, improving medical services work processes, and utilizing innovation for effective and patient-driven care. The idea of patient-focused care includes effectively including patients in their treatment choices, recognizing their inclinations and values, and advancing shared decision-production between medical services suppliers and patients.

Psychological wellness addresses a basic aspect in the talk on progressive treatment procedures. The worldwide commonness of emotional well-being conditions has arrived at disturbing levels, exacerbated by cultural tensions, monetary vulnerabilities, and the getting through shame encompassing psychological sickness. Traditional models of mental medical care frequently depend on drug mediations and psychotherapy, yet these methodologies miss the mark in giving exhaustive and open arrangements.

A progressive way to deal with emotional well-being includes destigmatizing psychological instabilities and incorporating psychological wellness into essential consideration. It requires a change in perspective towards preventive psychological well-being measures, early mediation, and the utilization of creative treatments. Innovation, including telemedicine and computerized therapeutics, can assume a critical part in extending admittance to emotional well-being administrations, especially in underserved or far off regions.

Besides, addressing the natural determinants of wellbeing is indispensable to progressive treatment methodologies. The 21st century is set apart by exceptional natural difficulties, including environmental change, contamination, and territory obliteration. These ecological variables in a roundabout way affect human wellbeing, adding to the spread of vector-borne sicknesses, respiratory diseases, and other medical problems.

Progressive treatment systems should recognize the association of human wellbeing and the climate. This includes advancing maintainable works on, moderating natural dangers, and integrating ecological contemplations into medical services strategies. The wellbeing area itself can add to natural supportability by embracing eco-accommodating works on, diminishing waste, and upholding for arrangements that focus on both human wellbeing and the prosperity of the planet.

Chapter 2

Understanding Cancer Biology

Understanding malignant growth science is a complicated and diverse undertaking that requires a complete investigation of the unpredictable components basic the turn of events and movement of this overwhelming sickness. Disease, at its center, is described by uncontrolled cell development and the capacity of these unusual cells to attack encompassing tissues, at last prompting the arrangement of threatening cancers. To unwind the secrets of malignant growth science, scientists dive into different angles, going from the hereditary and sub-atomic modifications driving tumorigenesis to the unpredictable exchange between the cancer microenvironment and the insusceptible framework.

One of the essential signs of disease is supported proliferative flagging, wherein disease cells secure the capacity to persistently develop and partition. This dysregulation frequently emerges from changes in qualities that control cell cycle movement, for example, those encoding cyclins, cyclin-subordinate kinases (CDKs), and cancer silencers like p53. These hereditary variations present a proliferative benefit to disease cells, permitting them to sidestep the ordinary administrative components that guarantee controlled cell division.

One more basic part of disease science is the avoidance of development silencers, a trademark that includes the disturbance of pathways answerable for restricting cell multiplication. Cancer silencer qualities, as p53 and retinoblastoma (RB), assume critical parts in limiting uncontrolled cell development. Loss-of-capability transformations in these qualities can release the proliferative capability of disease cells, adding to the persevering development of the growth mass.

Notwithstanding uncontrolled expansion, malignant growth cells display an exceptional limit with regards to dodging cell passing, which is one more sign of disease science. Apoptosis, a firmly managed course of modified cell demise, fills in as a pivotal component to dispense with harmed or undesirable cells. Nonetheless, disease cells frequently obtain hereditary modifications that render them impervious to apoptosis, permitting them to continue and aggregate extra transformations.

Genomic unsteadiness, one more trademark, assumes a critical part in the development of disease. The gathering of hereditary adjustments, including transformations, chromosomal revisions, and aneuploidy, adds to the heterogeneity saw inside cancers. This hereditary variety gives a substrate to normal choice, empowering disease cells to get worthwhile characteristics that improve their endurance and development.

Angiogenesis, the development of fresh blood vessels, is a trademark that supports the high metabolic requests of quickly developing growths. Malignant growth cells invigorate the improvement of an organization of veins to guarantee a consistent stock of oxygen and supplements. This interaction is organized by a harmony between favorable to angiogenic and hostile to angiogenic factors, and its dysregulation can fuel growth movement.

The capacity of disease cells to attack encompassing tissues and metastasize to far off organs addresses an impressive test in malignant growth science. This obtrusive way of behaving is worked with by adjustments in cell bond atoms, extracellular lattice parts, and compounds that intercede tissue corruption. The metastatic spread of malignant growth cells essentially adds to the dreariness and mortality related with the illness.

The growth microenvironment, containing stromal cells, safe cells, veins, and extracellular network, assumes a urgent part in profoundly shaping the way of behaving of disease cells. Collaborations between disease cells and their microenvironment impact key cycles like angiogenesis, safe avoidance, and metastasis. Understanding the powerful crosstalk between malignant growth cells and their environmental factors is fundamental for creating designated helpful intercessions.

Propels in genomic advancements have changed our capacity to take apart the hereditary scene of disease. Enormous scope sequencing projects, like The Malignant growth Genome Map book (TCGA), have given far reaching indexes of hereditary adjustments across different disease types.

These endeavors have recognized intermittent changes, duplicate number varieties, and chromosomal adjustments that drive tumorigenesis, offering important bits of knowledge into the sub-atomic premise of disease.

The field of disease genomics has divulged the amazing heterogeneity that exists among individual cancers and, surprisingly, inside a similar growth. Intratumor heterogeneity represents a critical test for creating powerful treatments, as various subclones inside a cancer might show unmistakable medication responsive qualities and obstruction instruments. Understanding and focusing on this heterogeneity are basic for conceiving customized therapy procedures custom-made to the novel hereditary cosmetics of every patient's disease.

Epigenetic changes, which include adjustments to DNA and histones that direct quality articulation, likewise assume a crucial part in disease science. Variant DNA methylation, histone changes, and non-coding RNA articulation can prompt the quieting of growth silencer qualities or the actuation of oncogenes. Focusing on epigenetic dysregulation addresses a promising road for remedial mediation in malignant growth.

The resistant framework is a blade that cuts both ways in malignant growth science. On one hand, the invulnerable framework has the ability to perceive and wipe out malignant growth cells through an interaction known as immunosurveillance. Then again, disease cells can utilize different techniques to sidestep insusceptible identification, prompting safe break and growth movement. Immunotherapy, which outfits the force of the resistant framework to target malignant growth cells, has arisen as a notable methodology in disease treatment.

Designated spot inhibitors, a class of immunotherapeutic specialists, block inhibitory signs that stifle the movement of cytotoxic Lymphocytes, releasing a resistant reaction against malignant growth cells. This change in perspective in disease treatment has shown exceptional progress in various malignancies, featuring the capability of immunotherapy as an extraordinary technique. In any case, difficulties like obstruction systems and distinguishing prescient biomarkers for reaction remain areas of dynamic exploration.

The transaction among irritation and malignant growth has for some time been perceived, with constant irritation filling in as a main thrust in tumorigenesis. Fiery cytokines and invulnerable cells inside the growth microenvironment add to disease advancement and movement. Understanding the unpredictable connection among aggravation and disease science is critical for creating designated treatments that disturb supportive of tumorigenic provocative pathways.

Digestion is arising as a key member in malignant growth science, with modifications in cell digestion being a sign of disease. Disease cells show metabolic reinventing to satisfy the expanded energy needs connected with fast multiplication.

The Warburg impact, described by a shift towards vigorous glycolysis even within the sight of oxygen, is a notable metabolic transformation in disease cells. Focusing on metabolic weaknesses in malignant growth cells addresses a promising road for remedial turn of events.

Accuracy medication, otherwise called customized medication, expects to fit clinical medicines to the singular qualities of every patient, including their hereditary cosmetics, way of life, and climate. In malignant growth, accuracy medication includes distinguishing explicit hereditary changes driving a patient's cancer and choosing designated treatments that exploit these weaknesses. This approach holds extraordinary commitment for further developing treatment results and limiting incidental effects.

Fluid biopsy, a painless technique for recognizing flowing growth DNA (ctDNA) and other biomarkers in the blood, is a progressive device in disease diagnostics and observing. Fluid biopsies give constant data about cancer elements, hereditary adjustments, and therapy reaction. This approach can possibly change malignant growth care by empowering early location, checking treatment reaction, and identifying insignificant lingering sickness.

In spite of the critical advancement in understanding malignant growth science, challenges continue making an interpretation of these experiences into successful treatments. Drug opposition, an unavoidable issue in malignant growth treatment, can emerge through different systems, including hereditary transformations, versatile changes, and the development of safe subclones. Beating drug obstruction requires a more profound comprehension of the basic systems and the improvement of imaginative remedial methodologies.

Mix treatments, which include the synchronous focusing of numerous pathways or instruments, address a promising way to deal with defeating drug opposition and further developing treatment viability. Levelheaded plan of mix regimens requires a careful comprehension of the sub-atomic and cell processes driving malignant growth, as well as the ID of synergistic connections between various helpful specialists.

The improvement of preclinical models, for example, hereditarily designed mouse models and patient-determined xenografts, assumes a critical part in propelling comprehension we might interpret malignant growth science and testing novel remedial mediations. These models reiterate key parts of human disease, giving significant stages to concentrating on cancer inception, movement, and reaction to therapy. Deciphering discoveries from preclinical models to clinical applications is a complex yet fundamental stage in drug improvement.

Clinical preliminaries are the foundation of assessing the security and adequacy of new malignant growth medicines. These preliminaries, directed in stages, include thorough testing in human subjects to decide the ideal dose, survey aftereffects, and assess treatment results.

Taking part in clinical preliminaries is basic for propelling disease research and furnishing patients with admittance to creative treatments that may not be accessible through standard medicines.

Disease immunotherapy, with its exceptional triumphs in specific malignancies, has prodded endeavors to grow its pertinence to a more extensive range of tumors. Research is in progress to recognize new immunotherapeutic targets, refine existing treatment regimens, and foster mix treatments that improve the counter growth resistant reaction. Conquering difficulties, for example, insusceptible opposition and understanding the mind boggling transaction between the resistant framework and disease cells are pivotal for additional propelling immunotherapy.

All in all, understanding malignant growth science is a dynamic and developing field that traverses numerous disciplines, from sub-atomic and cell science to genomics, immunology, and then some. Disentangling the complexities of tumorigenesis, movement, and helpful opposition is a considerable errand that requires cooperation among researchers, clinicians, and scientists around the world. Progresses in innovation, for example, high-throughput sequencing, CRISPR-Cas9 quality altering, and single-cell examination, keep on driving the boondocks of malignant growth research, opening new roads for revelation and development.

As we develop how we might interpret the sub-atomic and cell underpinnings of malignant growth, the way to viable disease treatments becomes more clear. Accuracy medication, immunotherapy, designated treatments, and creative mix approaches hold guarantee for changing disease treatment and working on persistent results. The excursion towards overcoming malignant growth is progressing, and the aggregate endeavors of established researchers, combined with the strength of patients and their families, move us forward in the journey for an existence where disease is at this point not an impressive foe.

2.1 Basics of cancer biology and how cancer cells proliferate

Understanding the rudiments of malignant growth science is significant for disentangling the many-sided systems by which disease cells multiply and dodge typical administrative cycles. Malignant growth, described by uncontrolled cell development and the capacity of these unusual cells to attack encompassing tissues, is a mind boggling and multi-layered sickness with establishes profoundly implanted in the sub-atomic and cell scene.

At the center of malignant growth science is the dysregulation of typical cell cycle control components. The cell cycle, an exceptionally organized process, oversees the movement of a cell from its introduction to the world to division. Vital participants in this guideline incorporate cyclins, cyclin-subordinate kinases (CDKs), and cancer silencer qualities, for example, p53. Transformations in these qualities can upset the sensitive harmony between cell division and cell cycle capture, prompting uncontrolled expansion — a trademark component of disease.

The cell cycle is partitioned into particular stages, including G1 (hole 1), S (amalgamation), G2 (hole 2), and M (mitosis). In G1, cells get ready for DNA amalgamation, while the S stage includes the replication of DNA. G2 marks the time of groundwork for cell division, and M envelops the real cell division process. Designated spots, managed by different proteins, guarantee the devotion of each stage, forestalling the movement of harmed or deficiently recreated cells.

Cancer silencer qualities, for example, p53, go about as watchmen of the genome. At the point when DNA harm is distinguished, p53 organizes a progression of occasions prompting cell cycle capture, permitting the cell to fix the harm prior to continuing. In the event that the harm is unsalvageable, p53 can set off apoptosis, wiping out the compromised cell. Changes in p53 or different parts of the DNA harm reaction pathway can handicap these defensive components, adding to the endurance of cells with harmed DNA and advancing tumorigenesis.

One more basic part of disease cell expansion includes the avoidance of development silencers. Cancer silencer qualities like RB (retinoblastoma) additionally assume vital parts in hindering extreme cell development. RB manages the change from G1 to S stage by hindering the action of E2F record factors. Loss of RB capability, frequently because of changes or inactivation by oncoproteins, can release the cell cycle, permitting uncontrolled cell expansion — a trademark element of numerous malignant growths.

Apoptosis, a customized type of cell passing, goes about as a shield against the endurance of harmed or undesirable cells. Disease cells, notwithstanding, can procure the capacity to sidestep apoptosis, a trademark that further adds to their uncontrolled development. Bcl-2 family proteins, for instance, assume a focal part in managing apoptosis. Overexpression of hostile to apoptotic Bcl-2 proteins or downregulation of supportive of apoptotic individuals can shift the equilibrium for cell endurance, empowering malignant growth cells to oppose demise signals.

Genomic flimsiness is a trademark include that adds to the heterogeneity saw inside cancers. DNA changes, chromosomal improvements, and aneuploidy — strange chromosome numbers — add to the hereditary variety found in disease. Genomic shakiness gives a substrate to normal determination inside the cancer microenvironment, permitting disease cells to obtain favorable qualities that improve their endurance and development.

Angiogenesis, the most common way of framing fresh blood vessels, is fundamental for supporting the high metabolic requests of quickly developing growths. Malignant growth cells discharge favorable to angiogenic factors that invigorate the development of veins, guaranteeing a persistent stockpile of oxygen and supplements. Vascular endothelial development factor (VEGF) is a central participant in this cycle. Focusing on angiogenesis has turned into a remedial procedure, with hostile to angiogenic drugs intending to remove the blood supply to cancers and restrain their development.

Attack and metastasis address basic strides in malignant growth movement. The capacity of disease cells to attack encompassing tissues and spread to far off organs represents a huge test in malignant growth treatment. Cell bond particles, lattice metalloproteinases (MMPs), and changes in the extracellular network work with disease cell movement and attack. Understanding these cycles is fundamental for creating procedures to obstruct metastasis and improve the viability of disease treatments.

The growth microenvironment, a unique milieu of stromal cells, safe cells, veins, and extracellular framework, assumes an essential part in profoundly shaping the way of behaving of disease cells. Connections between disease cells and their microenvironment impact key cycles like angiogenesis, safe avoidance, and metastasis. Disease related fibroblasts, safe cells, and flagging particles inside the microenvironment make a strong specialty for cancer development and movement.

Propels in genomics have given exceptional bits of knowledge into the hereditary changes driving malignant growth. Enormous scope drives like The Malignant growth Genome Chart book (TCGA) have indexed hereditary changes across different disease types. These endeavors have recognized repetitive changes, duplicate number varieties, and chromosomal modifications that fuel tumorigenesis, offering a complete comprehension of the sub-atomic premise of disease.

The field of malignant growth genomics has revealed the amazing heterogeneity existing among individual cancers and, surprisingly, inside a similar cancer. Intratumor heterogeneity represents a critical test for creating compelling treatments, as various subclones inside a cancer might show unmistakable medication responsive qualities and opposition systems. Focusing on this heterogeneity is pivotal for concocting customized therapy procedures custom-made to the exceptional hereditary cosmetics of every patient's disease.

Epigenetic changes, including changes to DNA and histones that direct quality articulation, likewise assume a vital part in disease science. Deviant DNA methylation, histone adjustments, and non-coding RNA articulation can prompt the quieting of growth silencer qualities or the actuation of oncogenes. Epigenetic changes add to the pliancy and flexibility of malignant growth cells, impacting their reaction to ecological signals and helpful intercessions.

The resistant framework is a basic player in malignant growth reconnaissance, fit for perceiving and disposing of disease cells through a cycle known as immunosurveillance. Nonetheless, disease cells can foster techniques to sidestep resistant discovery, prompting safe break and growth movement. Immunotherapy, a progressive methodology in malignant growth therapy, outfits the force of the safe framework to target and kill disease cells.

Designated spot inhibitors, a class of immunotherapeutic specialists, block inhibitory signs that smother the action of cytotoxic Lymphocytes, releasing a safe reaction against disease cells. This change in perspective in disease treatment has shown exceptional outcome in different malignancies, featuring the capability of immunotherapy as an extraordinary system. Difficulties, for example, distinguishing prescient biomarkers and understanding obstruction components are areas of dynamic exploration in the field.

The exchange among irritation and disease has for some time been perceived, with persistent aggravation filling in as a main thrust in tumorigenesis. Provocative cytokines and safe cells inside the growth microenvironment add to disease improvement and movement. Understanding the perplexing connection among irritation and malignant growth science is essential for creating designated treatments that disturb supportive of tumorigenic fiery pathways.

Digestion is arising as a key participant in malignant growth science, with modifications in cell digestion being a sign of disease. Disease cells show metabolic re-inventing to satisfy the expanded energy needs connected with fast expansion. The Warburg impact, described by a shift towards vigorous glycolysis even within the sight of oxygen, is a notable metabolic transformation in malignant growth cells. Focusing on metabolic weaknesses in disease cells addresses a promising road for helpful turn of events.

Accuracy medication, otherwise called customized medication, expects to fit clinical medicines to the singular qualities of every patient, including their hereditary cosmetics, way of life, and climate. In disease, accuracy medication includes distinguishing explicit hereditary changes driving a patient's growth and choosing designated treatments that exploit these weaknesses. This approach holds extraordinary commitment for further developing treatment results and limiting secondary effects.

Fluid biopsy, a painless technique for identifying circling growth DNA (ctDNA) and other biomarkers in the blood, is a progressive device in disease diagnostics and checking. Fluid biopsies give constant data about growth elements, hereditary adjustments, and treatment reaction. This approach can possibly change malignant growth care by empowering early discovery, observing treatment reaction, and identifying negligible remaining illness.

Notwithstanding huge advancement in understanding malignant growth science, challenges continue making an interpretation of these experiences into viable treatments. Drug obstruction, an unavoidable issue in malignant growth treatment, can emerge through different systems, including hereditary transformations, versatile changes, and the development of safe subclones. Defeating drug obstruction requires a more profound comprehension of the fundamental instruments and the improvement of creative helpful methodologies.

Blend treatments, including the concurrent focusing of various pathways or components, address a promising way to deal with conquering drug obstruction and further developing treatment viability. Normal plan of blend regimens requires a careful comprehension of the sub-atomic and cell processes driving malignant growth, as well as the distinguishing proof of synergistic communications between various restorative specialists.

The improvement of preclinical models, for example, hereditarily designed mouse models and patient-determined xenografts, assumes a urgent part in propelling comprehension we might interpret disease science and testing novel restorative mediations. These models reiterate key parts of human disease, giving significant stages to concentrating on growth commencement, movement, and reaction to treatment. Deciphering discoveries from preclinical models to clinical applications is a complex yet fundamental stage in drug improvement.

Clinical preliminaries are the foundation of assessing the security and adequacy of new disease medicines. These preliminaries, directed in stages, include thorough testing in human subjects to decide the ideal dose, survey secondary effects, and assess treatment results. Partaking in clinical preliminaries is basic for propelling malignant growth research and furnishing patients with admittance to creative treatments that may not be accessible through standard medicines.

Disease immunotherapy, with its striking triumphs in specific malignancies, has prodded endeavors to extend its relevance to a more extensive range of tumors. Research is in progress to recognize new immunotherapeutic targets, refine existing treatment regimens, and foster blend treatments that upgrade the counter cancer resistant reaction. Conquering difficulties, for example, insusceptible opposition and understanding the intricate transaction between the resistant framework and disease cells are significant for additional propelling immunotherapy.

2.2 Explanation of common cancer types and their characteristics

An extensive comprehension of normal disease types and their qualities is fundamental for clinicians, specialists, and patients the same. Malignant growth is a heterogeneous infection, with each kind having interesting highlights connected with its starting point, conduct, and reaction to treatment. Investigating the complexities of explicit disease types reveals insight into the different scene of oncology and guides fitted ways to deal with conclusion and helpful mediation.

Bosom malignant growth, one of the most predominant tumors around the world, emerges from the cells of the bosom tissue. It shows critical heterogeneity, enveloping subtypes with particular sub-atomic and neurotic attributes. The two essential classifications are painless (in situ) and obtrusive bosom disease. Ductal carcinoma in situ (DCIS) addresses a painless structure, bound to the milk pipes, while obtrusive ductal carcinoma (IDC) is portrayed by the penetration of malignant growth cells into encompassing tissues. Subtypes, for example, HER2-positive and triple-negative bosom disease have explicit atomic markers that impact treatment methodologies.

Cellular breakdown in the lungs, famous for its high death rate, is extensively ordered into little cell cellular breakdown in the lungs (SCLC) and non-little cell cellular breakdown in the lungs (NSCLC). SCLC, albeit more uncommon, will in general be more forceful. NSCLC involves adenocarcinoma, squamous cell carcinoma, and enormous cell carcinoma. Smoking is a significant gamble factor for cellular breakdown in the lungs, and early identification is testing, frequently prompting determination at cutting edge stages. Designated treatments and immunotherapy have arisen as promising roads for treating explicit subtypes of cellular breakdown in the lungs.

Colorectal disease, influencing the colon or rectum, positions among the main sources of malignant growth related passings. Adenocarcinoma is the dominating histological sort, emerging from the glandular cells covering the colorectal mucosa. Colorectal disease frequently creates from harmless polyps, accentuating the meaning of standard screenings. The infection movement includes stages from confined growths to territorial lymph hub inclusion and far off metastasis. Careful resection, chemotherapy, and immunotherapy comprise essential treatment modalities.

Prostate disease, basically influencing the prostate organ in men, is described by the strange development of prostate cells. Adenocarcinoma is the transcendent histological sort, representing most of cases. Prostate-explicit antigen (public service announcement) screening supports early discovery, however its utility is bantered because of worries about overdiagnosis and overtreatment. Prostate malignant growth displays a range of conduct, going from lethargic, slow-developing cancers to forceful structures with a high metastatic potential.

Ovarian disease is famous for its asymptomatic nature in beginning phases, prompting late-stage analyze and less fortunate results. Epithelial ovarian disease is the most widely recognized type, starting from the cells covering the ovaries. Other subtypes incorporate microbe cell growths and sex line stromal cancers. Ovarian disease frequently gives obscure side effects, adding to its difficulties in early recognition. Careful debulking, chemotherapy, and designated treatments comprise the essential treatment modalities.

Pancreatic malignant growth, infamous for its forceful nature, emerges from the cells of the pancreas. Pancreatic ductal adenocarcinoma (PDAC) is the most widely recognized subtype, described by its quick movement and protection from treatment. Early side effects are frequently vague, adding to late-organize analyze. Careful resection offers the main opportunity for fix, yet many cases present at cutting edge stages. Blend chemotherapy regimens and arising designated treatments plan to further develop results for pancreatic malignant growth patients.

Leukemia, a hematologic danger, includes the uncontrolled multiplication of blood-framing cells, influencing the bone marrow and blood. Intense leukemia, set apart by the fast collection of youthful platelets, incorporates intense lymphoblastic leukemia (ALL) and intense myeloid leukemia (AML).

Ongoing leukemia, described by the slow expansion in mature platelets, envelops persistent lymphocytic leukemia (CLL) and constant myeloid leukemia (CML). Treatment approaches change, including chemotherapy, designated treatments, and immature microorganism transplantation.

Lymphoma, emerging from the lymphatic framework, contains Hodgkin lymphoma (HL) and non-Hodgkin lymphoma (NHL). HL is portrayed by the presence of Reed-Sternberg cells and incorporates subtypes like nodular sclerosis and blended cellularity. NHL is more different, incorporating subtypes like diffuse enormous B-cell lymphoma (DLBCL), follicular lymphoma, and mantle cell lymphoma. Immunotherapy, designated treatments, and undifferentiated cell transplantation have changed the treatment scene for lymphomas.

Melanoma, starting from shade delivering cells called melanocytes, is a sort of skin malignant growth. Openness to bright (UV) radiation is a significant gamble factor. Melanoma is infamous for its capability to metastasize and is arranged into shallow spreading melanoma, nodular melanoma, lentigo maligna melanoma, and acral lentiginous melanoma. Early location is basic, and careful extraction stays the essential treatment. Immunotherapy and designated treatments have shown surprising progress in cutting edge melanoma cases.

Gastrointestinal stromal cancers (Significances) are uncommon growths that emerge in the gastrointestinal plot, frequently in the stomach or small digestive tract. Substances commonly harbor changes in the Unit or PDGFRA qualities, and designated treatments, for example, imatinib have upset their treatment. Careful resection is the pillar for restricted infection, however repetitive or metastatic cases benefit from designated treatment.

Mind cancers, starting inside the cerebrum or spinal rope, incorporate gliomas, meningiomas, and medulloblastomas. Glioblastoma multiforme (GBM), a forceful type of glioma, is especially difficult because of its infiltrative nature. Meningiomas, emerging from the meninges, are by and large sluggish developing and frequently harmless. Medulloblastomas, happening in the cerebellum, principally influence youngsters. Therapy shifts in view of the cancer type, area, and grade, frequently including a medical procedure, radiation, and chemotherapy.

Thyroid malignant growth emerges from the thyroid organ, with papillary thyroid carcinoma being the most widely recognized subtype. Follicular thyroid carcinoma, medullary thyroid carcinoma, and anaplastic thyroid carcinoma comprise other subtypes. Separated thyroid malignant growths, including papillary and follicular carcinomas, have good results with high endurance rates. Medullary and anaplastic thyroid carcinomas, notwithstanding, are more forceful and convey a less fortunate forecast.

Cervical disease, starting from the cells of the cervix, is many times gone before by pre-destructive changes perceptible through Pap spreads. Human papillomavirus (HPV) contamination is a significant gamble factor for cervical disease.

Squamous cell carcinoma and adenocarcinoma are the two essential histological subtypes. Beginning phase cervical malignant growth is frequently reparable with medical procedure, while cutting edge cases might require radiation and chemotherapy.

Bladder disease, emerging from the cells coating the bladder, is frequently connected with openness to cancer-causing agents, like those tracked down in tobacco. Urothelial carcinoma is the most well-known histological subtype, and other subtypes incorporate squamous cell carcinoma and adenocarcinoma. Treatment includes careful resection, intravesical treatment, and fundamental chemotherapy, with results changing in view of the stage and grade of the illness.

Endometrial malignant growth, influencing the covering of the uterus, is frequently connected to hormonal awkward nature, especially estrogen abundance. Endometrioid adenocarcinoma is the most well-known subtype, while other subtypes incorporate serous carcinoma and clear cell carcinoma. Endometrial malignant growth is frequently analyzed at a beginning phase, with medical procedure being the essential therapy. Adjuvant treatment might be suggested in light of the gamble factors.

Esophageal disease, emerging from the cells covering the throat, incorporates adenocarcinoma and squamous cell carcinoma subtypes. Gastroesophageal intersection (GEJ) disease, happening at the intersection of the throat and stomach, is likewise viewed as a kind of esophageal malignant growth. Risk factors incorporate smoking, liquor utilization, and gastroesophageal reflux sickness (GERD). Therapy includes a medical procedure, chemotherapy, and radiation, with results relying upon the stage and histological subtype.

Hepatocellular carcinoma (HCC), the essential type of liver malignant growth, frequently creates in the setting of ongoing liver illness, especially cirrhosis. Risk factors incorporate hepatitis B and C contaminations, liquor misuse, and non-alcoholic greasy liver illness (NAFLD). Careful resection, liver transplantation, and locoregional treatments are utilized for beginning phase illness, while fundamental treatments are utilized for cutting edge cases.

Renal cell carcinoma (RCC), the most widely recognized sort of kidney malignant growth, begins in the cells covering the renal tubules. Clear cell carcinoma is the overwhelming histological subtype, trailed by papillary and chromophobe carcinomas. Risk factors incorporate smoking, heftiness, and certain hereditary disorders. Careful resection is the pillar for limited sickness, while designated treatments and immunotherapy have further developed results for metastatic RCC.

Delicate tissue sarcomas envelop a different gathering of malignant growths emerging from delicate tissues, like muscles, ligaments, and fat. Subtypes incorporate liposarcoma, leiomyosarcoma, and synovial sarcoma.

Delicate tissue sarcomas can happen at whatever stage in life and may present as easy masses. Careful resection is the essential therapy, frequently supplemented by radiation and, now and again, fundamental treatment.

2.3 Overview of traditional cancer treatment methods and their limitations

An outline of conventional disease therapy strategies uncovers a multi-layered approach that incorporates a medical procedure, radiation treatment, and chemotherapy. While these techniques have been the pillar of disease treatment for a long time, they accompany innate limits that highlight the continuous requirement for creative and designated remedial methodologies.

Medical procedure, a basic part of disease therapy, includes the actual expulsion of growths or destructive tissues. It is many times the essential choice for limited and strong cancers that are agreeable to extraction. Careful mediations shift from insignificantly intrusive systems, like laparoscopy, to broad open medical procedures for bigger growths. While medical procedure can be corrective for some beginning phase diseases, its adequacy lessens when growths are broad or have metastasized.

One impediment of medical procedure lies in its failure to successfully address spread illness. In situations where malignant growth has spread to numerous locales or organs, complete annihilation through medical procedure becomes unfeasible. Furthermore, the obtrusiveness of a few surgeries might bring about confusions, expanded recuperation periods, and a diminished personal satisfaction for patients.

Radiation treatment utilizes ionizing radiation to target and annihilate malignant growth cells or hinder their capacity to isolate. A restricted therapy can be conveyed remotely (outer pillar radiation) or inside (brachytherapy). Radiation is successful in contracting cancers, diminishing side effects, and forestalling nearby repeat. In any case, its accuracy is significant, as neighboring sound tissues can likewise be impacted, prompting blow-back and possible aftereffects.

One impediment of radiation treatment is its limited reach, making it appropriate for the most part for restricted growths. Troubles emerge while managing dispersed or metastatic malignant growths, as lighting numerous destinations might bring about unreasonable poisonousness. Additionally, a tumors might display protection from radiation, restricting its viability in specific cases. The drawn out impacts of radiation, including the potential for optional malignant growths, highlight the significance of refining and advancing this therapy methodology.

Chemotherapy includes the utilization of medications that target quickly separating cells, including disease cells. It tends to be directed orally or intravenously and is many times used to treat fundamental or metastatic diseases.

Chemotherapy means to annihilate disease cells all through the body however is related with aftereffects because of its effect on common, solid cells with high turnover rates, like those in the bone marrow, gastrointestinal plot, and hair follicles.

The constraints of chemotherapy are clear in its vague nature, making harm solid tissues and bringing about unfriendly impacts like queasiness, weariness, going bald, and immunosuppression. Furthermore, the improvement of medication obstruction is a critical test, as malignant growth cells can adjust and develop to endure the cytotoxic impacts of chemotherapy. Blend chemotherapy regimens have been utilized to address opposition, yet this approach might prompt expanded poisonousness.

Chemical treatment is a designated approach that slows down the hormonal flagging pathways filling specific diseases. It is normally utilized in the therapy of chemical receptor-positive bosom and prostate malignant growths. By hindering chemical receptors or lessening chemical creation, this treatment plans to deny disease cells of the upgrades they need to develop. While chemical treatment can be viable, its pertinence is restricted to chemical delicate malignant growths, and opposition might foster over the long run.

Immunotherapy addresses a progressive change in disease therapy, outfitting the body's resistant framework to perceive and take out malignant growth cells. Designated spot inhibitors, monoclonal antibodies, and assenting cell treatments are among the immunotherapeutic methodologies acquiring noticeable quality. These therapies intend to conquer invulnerable avoidance components utilized by disease cells and upgrade the body's inherent capacity to target and obliterate them.

In spite of the astounding achievements of immunotherapy in specific tumors, it isn't generally compelling. Reaction rates differ among patients and disease types, and not all people show strong reactions. Recognizing prescient biomarkers and understanding the perplexing connections inside the cancer microenvironment are progressing difficulties in advancing the utilization of immunotherapy.

Designated treatment centers around unambiguous atomic pathways or proteins pivotal for disease cell endurance and development. Dissimilar to customary chemotherapy, which influences quickly partitioning cells unpredictably, designated treatments plan to restrain disease explicit targets specifically. Models incorporate tyrosine kinase inhibitors, chemical receptor blockers, and monoclonal antibodies. While designated treatments have shown viability as a rule, challenges emerge from the improvement of opposition and the requirement for persistent treatment.

Angiogenesis inhibitors address one more designated approach, expecting to disturb the development of fresh blood vessels that help cancer development. Drugs like bevacizumab target vascular endothelial development factor (VEGF), a central member in angiogenesis.

While these inhibitors have shown viability, obstruction systems and possible secondary effects, including hypertension and disabled injury mending, are significant contemplations.

Adjuvant and neoadjuvant treatments supplement essential medicines like a medical procedure and mean to upgrade their viability. Adjuvant treatment is controlled after the essential therapy to destroy lingering disease cells and decrease the gamble of repeat. Neoadjuvant treatment is given before the essential treatment, frequently to recoil cancers and work with careful resection. While these methodologies have further developed results as a rule, not all patients benefit, and the gamble of overtreatment stays a worry.

Restrictions in the conventional strategies for disease treatment feature the requirement for a more nuanced and customized approach. Accuracy medication, including designated treatments, immunotherapy, and genomic profiling, looks to tailor therapies in view of the particular hereditary and atomic qualities of every patient's disease. By distinguishing hereditary changes, adjustments, and biomarkers, accuracy medication expects to enhance remedial techniques, further develop reaction rates, and limit incidental effects.

Challenges in carrying out accuracy medication incorporate the intricacy of disease hereditary qualities, the advancing scene of obstruction components, and the requirement for powerful biomarkers. Also, admittance to cutting edge genomic profiling advances and the combination of huge scope information in clinical dynamic present calculated and down to earth difficulties.

The idea of blend treatments has gotten forward movement, including the concurrent utilization of various treatment modalities to accomplish synergistic impacts. Mixes might incorporate conventional medicines with immunotherapy, designated treatments, or other inventive methodologies. While promising, planning successful mix regimens requires a profound comprehension of the fundamental science of explicit diseases, possible cooperations, and the administration of expanded harmfulness.

The developing field of oncolytic infections addresses a clever remedial road. These infections are designed or normally happening to specifically taint and annihilate disease cells, while saving typical cells. Oncolytic infections invigorate an insusceptible reaction, further adding to their enemy of disease impacts. Clinical preliminaries investigating the security and adequacy of oncolytic infections, including herpes simplex infection and adenovirus-based vectors, are in progress.

Nanotechnology is likewise arising as a promising boondocks in disease treatment. Nanoparticles can be intended to convey helpful specialists straightforwardly to disease cells, upgrading drug conveyance and limiting foundational poisonousness. This approach holds potential for designated drug conveyance, imaging, and analytic applications. Nonetheless, challenges in nanoparticle solidness, leeway, and off-target impacts still need to be tended to.

Disease antibodies, including preventive immunizations for infection related malignant growths and helpful antibodies to invigorate the insusceptible framework against existing cancers, are being scrutinized. The advancement of viable disease immunizations faces obstacles connected with cancer heterogeneity, safe avoidance systems, and the distinguishing proof of reasonable antigens. By and by, propels in this field might add to the anticipation and therapy of explicit diseases.

Malignant growth undifferentiated organism treatment addresses a developing methodology focusing on the subpopulation of cells inside cancers that display foundational microorganism like properties. These cells are remembered to drive growth inception, movement, and protection from treatment. Creating procedures to specifically target and dispose of malignant growth undifferentiated organisms is a focal point of progressing research, determined to forestall backslide and working on long haul results.

Disease therapy techniques have gone through huge headways throughout the long term, enveloping a range of approaches pointed toward focusing on and wiping out malignant growth cells. These techniques principally incorporate a medical procedure, radiation treatment, chemotherapy, chemical treatment, immunotherapy, designated treatment, and a scope of arising and inventive methodologies. Every one of these modalities, while adding to the general advancement in disease treatment, conveys inborn limits that require a nuanced understanding and consistent investigation of novel remedial roads.

Medical procedure stays a foundation in the therapy of different tumors, especially those that are limited and strong in nature. The essential goal of careful mediation is the actual evacuation of growths or destructive tissues to accomplish a corrective result. Specialists might utilize negligibly intrusive methods, like laparoscopy, or select open medical procedures relying upon the nature and area of the growth. While medical procedure is frequently powerful for beginning phase tumors, its restrictions become obvious while managing broad or metastatic sickness.

The powerlessness of medical procedure to address dispersed malignant growth really represents a huge limit. In situations where malignant growth has spread to different organs or far off destinations, complete destruction through careful means becomes unfeasible. Moreover, the obtrusiveness of specific surgeries can bring about inconveniences, broadened recuperation periods, and a lessened personal satisfaction for patients. The limits of a medical procedure highlight the significance of coordinating other therapy modalities, particularly for diseases with fundamental inclusion.

Radiation treatment, using ionizing radiation to target and annihilate disease cells, addresses one more ordinary methodology in malignant growth therapy. This confined treatment can be directed remotely, known as outer shaft radiation, or inside through brachytherapy.

While radiation is viable in contracting growths and forestalling neighborhood repeat, it presents difficulties because of its vague nature, influencing close by sound tissues and causing blow-back.

The constraints of radiation treatment lie in its confined reach, delivering it generally appropriate for treating limited cancers. Troubles emerge while managing spread or metastatic malignant growths, as lighting various locales might prompt inordinate poisonousness. Besides, certain malignant growths might show protection from radiation, restricting its viability in those cases. Long haul impacts, including the potential for optional diseases, require a cautious harmony between accomplishing remedial advantages and limiting unfriendly outcomes.

Chemotherapy, a fundamental therapy including the organization of medications that target quickly isolating cells, has been a longstanding and broadly involved technique in malignant growth care. Chemotherapy can be conveyed orally or intravenously and is especially successful for treating foundational or metastatic malignant growths. In any case, its effect reaches out past malignant growth cells, influencing ordinary, solid cells with high turnover rates, prompting a scope of incidental effects.

The vague idea of chemotherapy is a huge limit, as it makes harm quickly separating sound cells in the bone marrow, gastrointestinal plot, and hair follicles, bringing about unfriendly impacts like sickness, exhaustion, balding, and immunosuppression. Furthermore, the improvement of medication obstruction represents a significant test, as disease cells can adjust and develop to endure the cytotoxic impacts of chemotherapy. Blend chemotherapy regimens have been utilized to address obstruction, however this approach might prompt expanded harmfulness.

Chemical treatment is a designated approach normally utilized in the therapy of chemical receptor-positive bosom and prostate malignant growths. This treatment plans to obstruct hormonal flagging pathways that fuel specific tumors, impeding chemical receptors or lessening chemical creation. While chemical treatment can be compelling, its pertinence is restricted to chemical delicate malignant growths, and obstruction might foster over the long run.

Immunotherapy, addressing a momentous change in perspective in disease therapy, use the body's resistant framework to perceive and take out malignant growth cells. Designated spot inhibitors, monoclonal antibodies, and supportive cell treatments are among the immunotherapeutic methodologies acquiring noticeable quality. These therapies intend to beat resistant avoidance systems utilized by malignant growth cells and upgrade the body's inherent capacity to target and obliterate them.

In spite of the surprising accomplishments of immunotherapy in specific tumors, its viability isn't general. Reaction rates differ among patients and malignant growth types, and not all people display strong reactions.

Distinguishing prescient biomarkers and understanding the perplexing connections inside the growth microenvironment are continuous difficulties in enhancing the utilization of immunotherapy. Moreover, insusceptible related antagonistic occasions and the potential for hyperactivation of the invulnerable framework require cautious observing and the executives.

Designated treatment centers around unambiguous atomic pathways or proteins vital for disease cell endurance and development. Dissimilar to customary chemotherapy, which influences quickly isolating cells unpredictably, designated treatments intend to hinder disease explicit targets specifically. Models incorporate tyrosine kinase inhibitors, chemical receptor blockers, and monoclonal antibodies. While designated treatments have shown viability as a rule, challenges emerge from the improvement of opposition and the requirement for persistent treatment.

Angiogenesis inhibitors address one more designated approach, meaning to upset the development of fresh blood vessels that help cancer development. Drugs like bevacizumab target vascular endothelial development factor (VEGF), a central participant in angiogenesis. While these inhibitors have shown adequacy, opposition instruments and possible secondary effects, including hypertension and weakened injury recuperating, are significant contemplations.

Adjuvant and neoadjuvant treatments supplement essential medicines like a medical procedure and mean to improve their viability. Adjuvant treatment is regulated after the essential therapy to destroy leftover disease cells and diminish the gamble of repeat. Neoadjuvant treatment is given before the essential treatment, frequently to shrivel cancers and work with careful resection. While these methodologies have further developed results generally speaking, not all patients benefit, and the gamble of overtreatment stays a worry.

Accuracy medication, enveloping designated treatments, immunotherapy, and genomic profiling, looks to tailor therapies in light of the particular hereditary and atomic attributes of every patient's malignant growth. By recognizing hereditary changes, adjustments, and biomarkers, accuracy medication intends to upgrade helpful procedures, further develop reaction rates, and limit aftereffects. Challenges in executing accuracy medication incorporate the intricacy of disease hereditary qualities, the advancing scene of obstruction systems, and the requirement for vigorous biomarkers.

The idea of blend treatments includes the concurrent utilization of various treatment modalities to accomplish synergistic impacts. Blends might incorporate conventional medicines with immunotherapy, designated treatments, or other imaginative methodologies. While promising, planning viable mix regimens requires a profound comprehension of the basic science of explicit diseases, possible cooperations, and the administration of expanded poisonousness.

Oncolytic infections, designed or normally happening to specifically contaminate and obliterate disease cells, address a clever restorative road. These infections invigorate an insusceptible reaction, further adding to their enemy of disease impacts. Clinical preliminaries investigating the security and viability of oncolytic infections, including herpes simplex infection and adenovirus-based vectors, are in progress. The improvement of oncolytic infections faces difficulties connected with growth heterogeneity, safe reactions, and streamlining their explicitness for disease cells.

Nanotechnology is arising as a promising outskirts in malignant growth therapy, with nanoparticles intended to convey remedial specialists straightforwardly to disease cells. This approach improves drug conveyance and limits foundational poisonousness. Challenges in nanoparticle soundness, freedom, and off-target impacts still need to be tended to, yet the potential for designated drug conveyance, imaging, and symptomatic applications is critical.

Malignant growth immunizations, both preventive and helpful, are being scrutinized as a way to forestall infection related diseases and invigorate the invulnerable framework against existing cancers. The improvement of viable disease antibodies faces obstacles connected with growth heterogeneity, invulnerable avoidance instruments, and the ID of appropriate antigens. Progresses in this field might add to the anticipation and therapy of explicit malignant growths.

Malignant growth foundational microorganism treatment is a developing methodology focusing on the subpopulation of cells inside cancers that show undifferentiated organism like properties. These cells are remembered to drive growth inception, movement, and protection from treatment. Creating procedures to specifically target and kill malignant growth foundational microorganisms is a focal point of progressing research, determined to forestall backslide and working on long haul results.

Chapter 3

Targeted Therapies

Designated treatments have arisen as a huge headway in the field of medication, offering more exact and successful medicines for different illnesses. Dissimilar to customary methodologies that frequently influence both sound and sick cells, designated treatments intend to focus on the basic sub-atomic components liable for a specific condition explicitly. This customized approach has shown promising outcomes in the therapy of malignant growth, immune system issues, and different sicknesses, upsetting the scene of present day medication.

In the domain of disease therapy, designated treatments have acquired noticeable quality for their capacity to impede explicit atoms associated with the development and endurance of malignant growth cells. Customary chemotherapy, while successful, can make huge harm sound cells, prompting different secondary effects. Designated treatments, then again, are intended to obstruct the signs that empower disease cells to develop and partition, saving typical cells from the horrendous impacts of treatment.

One of the critical highlights of designated treatments is the distinguishing proof of explicit sub-atomic focuses on that assume a urgent part in the turn of events and movement of sicknesses. In malignant growth, these objectives might incorporate proteins, receptors, or different particles that are overexpressed or transformed in disease cells. By pinpointing these objectives, specialists and clinicians can foster medications that specifically follow up on the strange cells, limiting harm to sound tissues.

With regards to malignant growth, the advancement of designated treatments has been especially groundbreaking. A change in outlook from the conventional one-size-fits-all way to deal with a more customized and exact treatment system has occurred. This shift is established in a more profound comprehension of the hereditary and sub-atomic changes that drive disease improvement. With headways in genomics and sub-atomic science, researchers can now portray the particular hereditary transformations and modifications present in individual growths, preparing for designated mediations.

One of the spearheading instances of designated treatments in malignant growth is the utilization of tyrosine kinase inhibitors (TKIs). Tyrosine kinases are chemicals that assume a critical part in the transmission of signs inside cells, impacting different cell processes, including cell development and endurance. In specific diseases, like ongoing myeloid leukemia (CML) and a few sorts of cellular breakdown in the lungs, explicit tyrosine kinases are unusually enacted, adding to the uncontrolled development of malignant growth cells.

Imatinib, a tyrosine kinase inhibitor, was perhaps the earliest designated treatment to exhibit momentous outcome in the treatment of CML. By specifically hindering the movement of the BCR-ABL tyrosine kinase, which is normal for CML, imatinib successfully actuates reduction in numerous patients. The outcome of imatinib established the groundwork for the improvement of another class of anticancer medications focusing on unambiguous sub-atomic anomalies.

Notwithstanding tyrosine kinase inhibitors, different classes of designated treatments have been created to address different atomic targets. Monoclonal antibodies, for example, are designed proteins that can tie to explicit focuses on the outer layer of disease cells, checking them for annihilation by the safe framework. Rituximab, utilized in the treatment of particular kinds of lymphoma, is an illustration of a monoclonal immune response that objectives the CD20 protein on B cells.

The progress of designated treatments in disease has enlivened scientists to investigate comparative methodologies in other clinical fields. Immune system sicknesses, described by an overactive safe reaction focusing on the body's own tissues, have turned into a concentration for designated treatment improvement. In conditions like rheumatoid joint pain and psoriasis, where explicit resistant pathways are dysregulated, drugs focusing on key atoms in these pathways can assist with tweaking the safe reaction and ease side effects.

Growth corruption factor (TNF) inhibitors, like infliximab and adalimumab, are instances of designated treatments utilized in immune system illnesses. These medications block the activity of TNF, a favorable to fiery cytokine that assumes a focal part in the pathogenesis of conditions like rheumatoid joint pain and provocative gut sickness. By killing TNF, these treatments assist with lessening irritation and slow the movement of the infections.

The outcome of designated treatments in malignant growth and immune system sicknesses has prompted their investigation in different regions, including irresistible illnesses and neurodegenerative problems. In irresistible sicknesses, the improvement of antiviral medications that explicitly target viral replication processes has demonstrated powerful in overseeing diseases like HIV and hepatitis C. Also, in nervous system science, the distinguishing proof of explicit sub-atomic targets related with neurodegenerative circumstances has provoked the examination of designated treatments for illnesses like Alzheimer's and Parkinson's.

The coming of accuracy medication, empowered by designated treatments, has introduced another time of medical services. This approach thinks about individual changeability in qualities, climate, and way of life, considering more customized and successful medicines. Hereditary testing and sub-atomic profiling assume a significant part in recognizing the particular irregularities driving a patient's sickness, directing clinicians in choosing the most suitable designated treatment.

Regardless of the astounding progress of designated treatments, difficulties and restrictions exist. One huge test is the improvement of protection from these treatments after some time. Disease cells, specifically, can advance and adjust, gaining changes that render designated treatments less compelling. This requires continuous exploration to figure out the instruments of obstruction and foster systems to survive or forestall it.

One more test is the ID of appropriate sub-atomic focuses for specific infections. Not all conditions have clear cut atomic targets, making it hard to foster designated treatments. Furthermore, the heterogeneity of sicknesses, especially in malignant growth, represents a test in recognizing a solitary objective that can successfully treat all patients with a particular kind of disease.

The expense of designated treatments is another variable that raises concerns. These medications frequently include mind boggling and modern assembling processes, adding to their significant expenses. Admittance to designated treatments can be restricted, particularly in locales with monetary requirements or where medical care frameworks might confront hardships in covering the costs related with these high level therapies.

Moral contemplations additionally become possibly the most important factor in the domain of designated treatments, especially with regards to hereditary testing.

The data got from hereditary testing brings up issues about protection, assent, and the potential for separation in light of hereditary inclinations. Finding some kind of harmony between propelling clinical information and safeguarding people's freedoms and security stays a basic thought.

Looking forward, continuous examination keeps on investigating new roads and refine existing designated treatments. Consolidating different designated specialists or incorporating them with customary treatment modalities is an area of dynamic examination. Combinatorial methodologies intend to upgrade treatment adequacy, defeat obstruction, and work on generally speaking patient results.

The field of immunotherapy addresses a promising boondocks in designated disease treatment. Immunotherapeutic methodologies tackle the force of the invulnerable framework to perceive and dispense with disease cells. Insusceptible designated spot inhibitors, for instance, block inhibitory signs that malignant growth cells use to sidestep discovery by the safe framework. These inhibitors have shown great outcomes in different malignant growths, including melanoma and particular kinds of cellular breakdown in the lungs.

The improvement of Vehicle Lymphocyte treatment is one more pivotal headway in malignant growth immunotherapy. Illusory Antigen Receptor Immune system microorganism treatment includes designing a patient's own Lymphocytes to communicate receptors that target explicit proteins on the outer layer of malignant growth cells. This customized approach has shown momentous progress in the treatment of specific hematologic malignancies, for example, intense lymphoblastic leukemia.

In the domain of irresistible sicknesses, the improvement of antiviral treatments keeps on advancing. The continuous danger of arising infections, as featured by the Coronavirus pandemic, highlights the significance of designated antiviral methodologies. Scientists are investigating drugs that explicitly restrain viral replication processes, offering an additional designated and powerful method for overseeing viral diseases.

Neurological issues, with their mind boggling and multifactorial nature, present interesting difficulties for designated treatment improvement. In any case, progressing research is uncovering potential atomic targets related with conditions like Alzheimer's and Parkinson's. Focusing on unambiguous pathways engaged with neurodegeneration might offer new roads for easing back or stopping infection movement.

All in all, designated treatments address an extraordinary power in present day medication, offering more exact and compelling medicines across a range of illnesses. From the early triumphs in malignant growth therapy with tyrosine kinase inhibitors to the venture into immune system sicknesses, irresistible illnesses, and neurodegenerative problems, designated treatments have reshaped the scene of clinical consideration.

The continuous refinement of these treatments, combined with progresses in genomics, sub-atomic science, and immunology, holds the commitment of additional forward leaps. As scientists dig further into the atomic underpinnings of sicknesses, new and more unambiguous targets will probably arise, making ready for the improvement of progressively customized and customized therapy systems.

3.1 Introduction to targeted therapies and their potential

Designated treatments address a progressive methodology in the field of medication, offering a more exact and centered strategy for treating different sicknesses. Not at all like customary medicines that frequently influence both solid and sick cells, designated treatments expect to address the hidden sub-atomic instruments liable for a specific condition explicitly. This approach has shown critical commitment in the therapy of malignant growth, immune system issues, and different sicknesses, in a general sense changing the scene of current clinical practices.

The focal precept of designated treatments lies in their capacity to recognize and specifically address explicit sub-atomic targets related with a given illness. With regards to disease, for instance, these objectives might incorporate proteins, receptors, or different particles that are either overexpressed or changed in malignant growth cells. The goal is to pinpoint these unusual components and foster medications that demonstration with accuracy, limiting inadvertent blow-back to solid tissues and cells.

The coming of designated treatments has especially changed malignant growth treatment, giving a takeoff from the traditional one-size-fits-all methodology. Conventional chemotherapy, while powerful, can hurt solid cells, prompting a horde of secondary effects. Interestingly, designated treatments center around upsetting the signs that fuel the development and endurance of malignant growth cells, offering a more custom fitted and less harmful intercession.

A perfect representation of designated treatments in disease is the utilization of tyrosine kinase inhibitors (TKIs). Tyrosine kinases are proteins pivotal for sending signals inside cells, impacting cycles like cell development and endurance. In specific malignant growths, explicit tyrosine kinases are abnormally enacted, adding to the uncontrolled multiplication of disease cells. Imatinib, a trailblazer in this class of medications, has shown wonderful progress in treating ongoing myeloid leukemia (CML) by restraining the BCR-ABL tyrosine kinase normal for CML cells.

The outcome of imatinib has made ready for the improvement of a more extensive range of designated treatments in disease. Monoclonal antibodies, one more class of designated treatments, are designed proteins intended to tie to explicit focuses on the outer layer of disease cells, stamping them for annihilation by the safe framework.

Rituximab, utilized in specific kinds of lymphoma, represents the adequacy of monoclonal antibodies by focusing on the CD20 protein on B cells.

The designated treatment worldview has not been restricted to disease alone. Immune system sicknesses, portrayed by an overactive invulnerable reaction focusing on the body's own tissues, have turned into a point of convergence for designated treatment improvement. Conditions like rheumatoid joint pain and psoriasis, where explicit resistant pathways are dysregulated, have seen the appearance of medications focusing on key atoms in these pathways to tweak the safe reaction and mitigate side effects.

TNF inhibitors, like infliximab and adalimumab, stand apart as instances of designated treatments utilized in immune system illnesses. By obstructing the activity of cancer rot factor (TNF), a favorable to fiery cytokine vital to the pathogenesis of infections like rheumatoid joint pain and provocative inside sickness, these treatments really decrease irritation and block illness movement.

The outcome of designated treatments in malignant growth and immune system sicknesses has prodded investigation into their application in other clinical areas. Irresistible sicknesses, for example, have seen the improvement of antiviral medications that explicitly target viral replication processes, demonstrating powerful in overseeing diseases like HIV and hepatitis C. Essentially, in nervous system science, the ID of explicit atomic targets related with neurodegenerative circumstances has provoked the examination of designated treatments for illnesses like Alzheimer's and Parkinson's.

Accuracy medication, supported by designated treatments, denotes a change in perspective in medical care. This approach considers individual changeability in qualities, climate, and way of life, taking into consideration more customized and compelling medicines. Hereditary testing and sub-atomic profiling assume urgent parts in recognizing the particular hereditary transformations and modifications that drive a patient's sickness, directing clinicians in choosing the most proper designated treatment.

Regardless of the astounding steps in designated treatment advancement, difficulties and restrictions persevere. One of the critical provokes is the development of protection from these treatments over the long run. Malignant growth cells, specifically, can develop and adjust, procuring changes that render designated treatments less viable. Understanding the instruments of opposition and creating techniques to survive or forestall it stay dynamic areas of examination.

Recognizing appropriate atomic focuses for specific sicknesses represents another test. Not all conditions have clear cut atomic targets, making it challenging to foster designated treatments.

The heterogeneity of sicknesses, particularly in disease, further convolutes the recognizable proof of a solitary objective that can successfully treat all patients with a particular sort of malignant growth.

The expense of designated treatments is a significant concern. The complex assembling processes associated with delivering these medications add to their significant expenses. Admittance to designated treatments can be restricted, especially in locales with monetary requirements or where medical care frameworks battle to cover the costs related with these high level therapies.

Moral contemplations likewise become possibly the most important factor, particularly with regards to hereditary testing. The data acquired from hereditary testing brings up issues about protection, assent, and the potential for segregation in view of hereditary inclinations. Finding some kind of harmony between propelling clinical information and safeguarding people's privileges and protection stays a basic thought.

Looking forward, progressing research plans to investigate new roads and refine existing designated treatments. Joining different designated specialists or incorporating them with conventional treatment modalities is a functioning area of examination. Combinatorial methodologies try to upgrade treatment viability, defeat opposition, and work on by and large persistent results.

Immunotherapy addresses an especially encouraging outskirts in designated disease treatment. Immunotherapeutic methodologies influence the safe framework to perceive and kill disease cells. Resistant designated spot inhibitors, for example, block inhibitory signs that disease cells exploit to avoid discovery by the invulnerable framework. These inhibitors have shown amazing outcomes in different tumors, including melanoma and specific sorts of cellular breakdown in the lungs.

The improvement of Vehicle Lymphocyte treatment remains as one more notable progression in disease immunotherapy. Illusory Antigen Receptor Lymphocyte treatment includes designing a patient's own Immune system microorganisms to communicate receptors that target explicit proteins on the outer layer of disease cells. This customized approach has shown striking outcome in treating specific hematologic malignancies, for example, intense lymphoblastic leukemia.

In irresistible illnesses, the advancement of antiviral treatments proceeds. The continuous danger of arising infections, as highlighted by the Coronavirus pandemic, accentuates the significance of designated antiviral methodologies. Specialists are investigating drugs that explicitly hinder viral replication processes, offering an additional designated and powerful method for overseeing viral contaminations.

Neurological problems present interesting moves for designated treatment improvement because of their perplexing and multifactorial nature. By and by, progressing research is uncovering potential sub-atomic targets related with conditions like Alzheimer's and Parkinson's. Focusing on unambiguous pathways engaged with neurodegeneration holds the commitment of opening new roads for easing back or ending infection movement.

All in all, designated treatments have arisen as a groundbreaking power in current medication, giving a more exact and viable way to deal with treating a wide exhibit of illnesses. From the early triumphs in malignant growth therapy with tyrosine kinase inhibitors to the venture into immune system sicknesses, irresistible illnesses, and neurodegenerative problems, designated treatments have reshaped the scene of clinical consideration.

As these treatments keep on being refined and extended, directed by propels in genomics, atomic science, and immunology, the potential for additional forward leaps stays high. More profound bits of knowledge into the atomic underpinnings of infections will probably uncover new and more unambiguous targets, preparing for the advancement of progressively custom-made and customized treatment systems.

In spite of the difficulties and moral contemplations, the effect of designated treatments on medical care is significant. The shift toward accuracy medication, driven by the standards of designated treatment, guarantees a future where medicines are more powerful as well as better lined up with the singular qualities of every patient. As the excursion of disclosure unfurls, the impact of designated treatments on human wellbeing is ready to arrive at extraordinary levels, offering trust and recuperating to people confronting different ailments.

3.2 Exploration of precision medicine and personalized treatment

The coming of accuracy medication denotes a groundbreaking change in perspective in medical care, proclaiming another time of customized therapy approaches custom-made to individual patients. Accuracy medication, otherwise called customized or individualized medication, underlines the customization of clinical consideration in light of the special qualities of every patient. This progressive idea use headways in genomics, atomic science, and innovation to figure out the hereditary and sub-atomic cosmetics of illnesses, preparing for additional designated and compelling mediations.

At the center of accuracy medication is the acknowledgment that people vary in their outward side effects as well as at the hereditary and sub-atomic levels. Conventional clinical methodologies frequently embrace a one-size-fits-all model, where medicines are normalized for a specific infection or condition. In any case, this approach neglects to represent the intrinsic changeability among patients, prompting varieties in treatment reactions and results.

Accuracy medication looks to address this impediment by considering the hereditary, natural, and way of life factors that add to a singular's wellbeing. The mix of genomic data into clinical practice has been a critical driver of accuracy medication. The Human Genome Venture, finished in 2003, assumed a critical part in planning the whole human genome, giving an exhaustive reference to grasping the hereditary premise of wellbeing and illness.

Genomic information, including data about a singular's DNA arrangement, quality articulation, and hereditary varieties, structure the groundwork of accuracy medication. The utilization of cutting edge sequencing innovations has empowered the fast and financially savvy examination of huge genomic datasets, working with a more profound comprehension of the hereditary elements hidden different sicknesses.

Disease has been an essential focal point of accuracy medication drives, given its perplexing and heterogeneous nature. The distinguishing proof of explicit hereditary transformations and modifications in disease cells has prepared for designated treatments that address the remarkable atomic drivers of every patient's malignant growth. Sub-atomic profiling of growths permits clinicians to decide the best therapy procedures, fitting mediations in light of the individual hereditary cosmetics of the disease.

One of the notable utilizations of accuracy medication in malignant growth is the utilization of designated treatments, like tyrosine kinase inhibitors (TKIs) and monoclonal antibodies. These treatments are intended to explicitly target sub-atomic irregularities present in malignant growth cells, limiting harm to typical cells and lessening aftereffects contrasted with conventional chemotherapy.

The progress of designated treatments in disease has motivated the investigation of accuracy medication in other clinical claims to fame. Immune system infections, portrayed by an overactive safe reaction focusing on the body's own tissues, have turned into a concentration for customized treatment methodologies. By understanding the particular safe pathways dysregulated in conditions like rheumatoid joint pain and lupus, scientists can foster designated treatments that tweak the resistant reaction with more prominent accuracy.

In irresistible sicknesses, accuracy medication has added to the improvement of antiviral treatments that explicitly focus on the replication cycles of infections. This designated approach has demonstrated successful in overseeing diseases like HIV and hepatitis C, offering an additional custom fitted and proficient method for treatment.

Neurological issues, with their complex and multifactorial nature, present exceptional difficulties for accuracy medication. In any case, continuous exploration is revealing explicit hereditary and sub-atomic targets related with conditions like Alzheimer's and Parkinson's illness. Accuracy medication holds the commitment of giving more successful medicines that address the basic reasons for neurodegenerative problems.

The mix of accuracy medication into clinical practice depends on the extensive investigation of patient information, including hereditary data, clinical history, and ecological variables. Electronic wellbeing records (EHRs) assume a critical part in this cycle by giving a unified storehouse of patient data open to medical care suppliers. The consistent trade of data between medical care frameworks works with an all encompassing comprehension of every patient's wellbeing, empowering more educated and customized therapy choices.

The ascent of accuracy medication has additionally prompted the development of interdisciplinary coordinated efforts between medical care experts, geneticists, bioinformaticians, and different specialists. The collaboration of assorted fields is fundamental for deciphering complex genomic information, making an interpretation of hereditary bits of knowledge into significant treatment procedures, and guaranteeing the moral and capable utilization of hereditary data.

In spite of the commitment and capability of accuracy medication, a few difficulties and moral contemplations continue. One of the essential difficulties is the translation of genomic information. The sheer volume and intricacy of hereditary data produced by sequencing advances require modern bioinformatics apparatuses and skill to remove significant bits of knowledge. Clinicians and scientists should explore the complexities of genomic information to recognize pertinent hereditary varieties and their suggestions for patient consideration.

One more test lies in the normalization and coordination of accuracy medication approaches into routine clinical practice. The execution of genomic testing and customized treatment methodologies requires cautious thought of administrative systems, moral rules, and the advancement of proof based rehearses. Guaranteeing evenhanded admittance to accuracy medication across different populaces is likewise a basic part of tending to medical care inconsistencies.

Moral contemplations assume a focal part in the capable execution of accuracy medication. Issues, for example, patient assent for hereditary testing, security of genomic data, and the potential for hereditary separation require cautious consultation. Finding some kind of harmony between propelling clinical information and safeguarding individual privileges and protection is vital for building trust in the utilization of accuracy medication.

The monetary ramifications of accuracy medication, incorporating the expenses related with genomic testing and customized medicines, are extra contemplations. While the diminishing expenses of genomic sequencing have made hereditary testing more available, the reasonableness and repayment of designated treatments remain difficulties. These financial variables can affect the far and wide reception of accuracy medication in medical services frameworks all around the world.

Regardless of these difficulties, the likely advantages of accuracy medication are monstrous. Fitting medicines in view of individual hereditary profiles can prompt more compelling mediations, less unfavorable impacts, and worked on understanding results. Moreover, the capacity to recognize people at higher gamble of specific infections considers preventive measures and early intercessions, changing medical services from a responsive to a proactive model.

The continuous development of accuracy medication includes progressions in innovation and logical comprehension as well as a change in the mentality of medical services suppliers, scientists, and the overall population. Embracing a patient-driven approach, accuracy medication underscores the significance of individualized care, perceiving that every patient is novel and may answer distinctively to explicit medicines.

As accuracy medication keeps on propelling, the field holds guarantee for tending to beforehand recalcitrant clinical difficulties. Uncommon illnesses, described by their hereditary premise and frequently ignored in customary medication advancement, stand to profit from the customized treatment approaches presented by accuracy medication. By understanding the particular hereditary changes answerable for interesting infections, scientists can foster designated treatments custom-made to the fundamental hereditary anomalies.

The reconciliation of computerized reasoning (man-made intelligence) and AI (ML) into accuracy medication further upgrades its abilities. These advances can break down tremendous measures of genomic and clinical information, recognize designs, and produce bits of knowledge that may not be evident through conventional techniques. Computer based intelligence and ML applications in accuracy medication can possibly speed up the speed of disclosure, advance treatment methodologies, and add to more customized and productive medical care conveyance.

All in all, accuracy medication addresses a progressive way to deal with medical services, underscoring customized therapy procedures in view of individual hereditary and sub-atomic profiles. From its beginnings in malignant growth therapy to its extending applications in immune system sicknesses, irresistible illnesses, and neurodegenerative problems, accuracy medication has reshaped the scene of clinical consideration.

As genomic innovations proceed to progress, and interdisciplinary coordinated efforts extend, the eventual fate of accuracy medication holds energizing prospects. The continuous refinement of genomic testing, designated treatments, and the moral systems encompassing accuracy medication will add to its consistent combination into routine clinical practice. The excursion towards accuracy medication connotes a shift towards more individualized, viable, and patient-driven medical services, offering new expectation and opportunities for the fate of medication.

3.3 Highlighting successful targeted therapy approaches

Designated treatments have arisen as a progressive methodology in the treatment of different illnesses, offering more exact and compelling mediations contrasted with customary medicines. The outcome of designated treatments lies in their capacity to target atomic irregularities that drive sickness movement, limiting harm to sound cells and lessening aftereffects explicitly. This segment investigates fruitful designated treatment approaches across various clinical spaces, highlighting their effect on quiet results.

In the domain of malignant growth therapy, designated treatments have exhibited exceptional accomplishment by tending to explicit atomic abnormalities present in disease cells. One of the spearheading models is the utilization of tyrosine kinase inhibitors (TKIs) in the therapy of ongoing myeloid leukemia (CML). Imatinib, an original TKI, focuses on the BCR-ABL tyrosine kinase, which is normal for CML cells. Imatinib has changed the anticipation for the majority CML patients, inciting reduction and fundamentally further developing long haul endurance rates.

The progress of TKIs reaches out past CML to different sorts of malignant growth, including non-little cell cellular breakdown in the lungs (NSCLC). EGFR (epidermal development factor receptor) transformations are predominant in NSCLC, and drugs like erlotinib and gefitinib explicitly focus on these changes. These EGFR inhibitors have exhibited adequacy in further developing movement free endurance and in general endurance in patients with EGFR-freak NSCLC.

One more eminent outcome in disease designated treatment is the utilization of monoclonal antibodies. Rituximab, a monoclonal neutralizer focusing on the CD20 protein on B cells, has demonstrated successful in the treatment of specific B-cell lymphomas. By restricting to CD20, rituximab triggers the insusceptible framework to perceive and annihilate dangerous B cells. This designated approach has altogether further developed results for patients with B-cell lymphomas.

In the domain of immune system sicknesses, designated treatments have altered the administration of conditions like rheumatoid joint pain (RA). Growth rot factor (TNF) inhibitors, including infliximab and adalimumab, have exhibited outcome in RA by obstructing the activity of TNF, a supportive of fiery cytokine ensnared in the pathogenesis of the sickness. These designated treatments assist with decreasing aggravation, ease side effects, and slow infection movement.

The outcome of TNF inhibitors in RA reaches out to other immune system conditions, like psoriasis and fiery entrail illness. Adalimumab, for instance, is endorsed for the treatment of psoriasis and has shown adequacy in actuating and keeping up with abatement in fiery gut sicknesses like Crohn's illness and ulcerative colitis.

In irresistible illnesses, especially with regards to viral contaminations, designated treatments have demonstrated powerful in overseeing sicknesses like HIV. Antiretroviral treatment (Workmanship) addresses a fruitful designated way to deal with hinder different phases of the HIV life cycle. Various classes of antiretroviral drugs target viral compounds, keeping the infection from duplicating and lessening the viral burden in patients with HIV. The coming of Craftsmanship has changed HIV from a hazardous condition to a sensible persistent illness.

The advancement of direct-acting antivirals (DAAs) addresses one more victory in designated treatment, particularly in the treatment of hepatitis C. DAAs explicitly target viral proteins fundamental for the replication of the hepatitis C infection. The presentation of DAAs has reformed the treatment scene for hepatitis C, offering high fix rates with more limited treatment terms and less secondary effects contrasted with past regimens.

In the area of nervous system science, designated treatments are acquiring conspicuousness in the treatment of neurodegenerative issues. Alzheimer's sickness, portrayed by the collection of beta-amyloid plaques in the mind, has seen the improvement of designated treatments planning to alter illness movement. Monoclonal antibodies like aducanumab have been intended to target and clear beta-amyloid plaques, addressing a clever way to deal with Alzheimer's illness treatment.

Parkinson's illness, a neurodegenerative issue described by the deficiency of dopamine-creating neurons, has likewise seen headways in designated treatments. Profound cerebrum excitement (DBS) is a careful mediation that includes embedding terminals in unambiguous mind locales and regulating their movement to lighten engine side effects related with Parkinson's illness. While not a pharmacological treatment, DBS represents the designated and customized nature of mediations in neurodegenerative issues.

The outcome of designated treatments in malignant growth has prompted imaginative methodologies, like immunotherapy. Resistant designated spot inhibitors, including drugs like pembrolizumab and nivolumab, have shown striking outcome in different diseases, including melanoma, cellular breakdown in the lungs, and renal cell carcinoma. These inhibitors block the inhibitory signs that disease cells exploit to dodge identification by the resistant framework, releasing the body's invulnerable reaction to target and kill malignant growth cells.

Illusory Antigen Receptor White blood cell treatment (Vehicle T treatment) addresses a momentous headway in malignant growth immunotherapy. This customized approach includes changing a patient's own Lymphocytes to communicate receptors focusing on unambiguous proteins on the outer layer of malignant growth cells. Vehicle T treatment has shown extraordinary progress in treating specific hematologic malignancies, especially intense lymphoblastic leukemia and non-Hodgkin lymphoma.

The outcome of designated treatments isn't exclusively ascribed to their adequacy yet in addition to the change in treatment ideal models they have catalyzed. The idea of accuracy medication, directed by the standards of designated treatment, stresses the customization of medicines in view of individual patient attributes. Genomic testing and sub-atomic profiling assume a critical part in distinguishing explicit hereditary transformations and atomic irregularities, directing clinicians in choosing the most suitable designated treatment for every patient.

In spite of the astounding victories, difficulties and contemplations exist in the domain of designated treatments. One critical test is the improvement of obstruction over the long haul. Malignant growth cells, specifically, can develop and adjust, gaining changes that render designated treatments less compelling. This requires continuous exploration to grasp the instruments of opposition and foster systems to survive or forestall it.

Distinguishing reasonable sub-atomic focuses for specific infections is another test. Not all conditions have distinct atomic targets, making it challenging to foster designated treatments. The heterogeneity of illnesses, especially in malignant growth, represents a test in recognizing a solitary objective that can really treat all patients with a particular sort of disease.

The expense of designated treatments is a component that raises concerns. These medications frequently include complex assembling processes, adding to their significant expenses. Admittance to designated treatments can be restricted, particularly in locales with monetary imperatives or where medical care frameworks might confront troubles in covering the costs related with these high level therapies.

Moral contemplations likewise become possibly the most important factor in the domain of designated treatments, especially with regards to hereditary testing. The data acquired from hereditary testing brings up issues about protection, assent, and the potential for separation in light of hereditary inclinations. Finding some kind of harmony between propelling clinical information and safeguarding people's freedoms and protection stays a basic thought.

Taking everything into account, the outcome of designated treatments across different clinical spaces features their extraordinary effect on persistent consideration. From the early accomplishments in malignant growth therapy with tyrosine kinase inhibitors and monoclonal antibodies to the progressions in immune system sicknesses, irresistible illnesses, and neurodegenerative issues, designated treatments have reshaped the scene of clinical mediations.

The excursion of designated treatments is set apart by development, accuracy, and a patient-driven approach. As scientists dig further into the sub-atomic underpinnings of illnesses, new and more unambiguous targets will probably arise, preparing for the advancement of progressively customized and customized treatment procedures.

Notwithstanding the difficulties and moral contemplations, the capability of designated treatments to change medical care couldn't possibly be more significant, offering trust and mending to people confronting a different cluster of ailments.

Designated treatment approaches have arisen as a progressive and exceptionally powerful methodology in the field of medication, offering an exact and customized method for treating a great many sicknesses. This extraordinary methodology includes the distinguishing proof and particular focusing of explicit particles or pathways engaged with the development and endurance of strange cells, for example, malignant growth cells or cells adding to immune system issues. The progress of designated treatments lies in their capacity to slow down the fundamental atomic components driving illness, while limiting harm to ordinary cells. This part investigates different designated treatment approaches across various clinical disciplines, exhibiting their critical effect on understanding results.

In disease treatment, one of the spearheading designated treatment approaches includes the utilization of tyrosine kinase inhibitors (TKIs). Tyrosine kinases are catalysts that assume a significant part in sending signals inside cells, impacting different cell processes, including cell development and endurance. Deviant enactment of tyrosine kinases is a typical element in numerous tumors. Imatinib, for example, has been exceptionally fruitful in treating constant myeloid leukemia (CML) by explicitly restraining the BCR-ABL tyrosine kinase normal for CML cells. The outcome of imatinib established the groundwork for the improvement of another class of designated treatments in malignant growth.

Monoclonal antibodies address one more class of designated treatments broadly utilized in disease treatment. These designed antibodies are intended to perceive and tie to explicit proteins on the outer layer of malignant growth cells. Rituximab, utilized in the treatment of specific B-cell lymphomas, focuses on the CD20 protein on B cells, stamping them for obliteration by the resistant framework. Trastuzumab, another monoclonal counter acting agent, focuses on the HER2 protein and has been fruitful in treating HER2-positive bosom disease.

Notwithstanding tyrosine kinase inhibitors and monoclonal antibodies, little particle inhibitors have demonstrated viable in malignant growth designated treatment. For instance, inhibitors of poly (ADP-ribose) polymerase (PARP) have shown outcome in the therapy of specific sorts of bosom and ovarian malignant growths, especially those with BRCA transformations. PARP inhibitors exploit lacks in DNA fix systems in disease cells, prompting their particular obliteration.

Immunotherapy has arisen as a weighty designated treatment approach in malignant growth treatment. Insusceptible designated spot inhibitors, for example, pembrolizumab and nivolumab, release the body's invulnerable framework to perceive and go after disease cells. These inhibitors block the inhibitory signs that disease cells exploit to dodge discovery by the resistant framework. Immunotherapy has exhibited huge progress in different malignant growths, including melanoma, cellular breakdown in the lungs, and renal cell carcinoma.

Fanciful Antigen Receptor Lymphocyte treatment (Vehicle T treatment) addresses a progressive customized way to deal with disease immunotherapy. This imaginative treatment includes changing a patient's own Lymphocytes to communicate receptors focusing on unambiguous proteins on the outer layer of disease cells. Vehicle T treatment has shown striking outcome in treating specific hematologic malignancies, including intense lymphoblastic leukemia and non-Hodgkin lymphoma.

In the field of immune system sicknesses, designated treatments have changed the administration of conditions described by dysregulated safe reactions. Growth putrefaction factor (TNF) inhibitors, including infliximab and adalimumab, have been effective in conditions like rheumatoid joint pain, psoriasis, and provocative gut illness. By impeding the activity of TNF, these treatments tweak the invulnerable reaction, diminishing aggravation and mitigating side effects.

Interleukin-17 (IL-17) inhibitors, for example, secukinumab and ixekizumab, address one more designated treatment approach in immune system sicknesses. These inhibitors explicitly target IL-17, a favorable to fiery cytokine ensnared in the pathogenesis of conditions like psoriasis and ankylosing spondylitis. By killing IL-17, these treatments assist with lightening side effects and work on the personal satisfaction for patients.

Janus kinase (JAK) inhibitors have arisen as a flexible class of designated treatments in immune system illnesses. Drugs like tofacitinib and baricitinib focus on the JAK-Detail flagging pathway, which assumes a focal part in safe reactions. These inhibitors have shown viability in conditions like rheumatoid joint pain and psoriatic joint inflammation, giving a designated way to deal with regulating resistant brokenness.

In irresistible sicknesses, especially with regards to viral diseases, designated treatments have demonstrated powerful in overseeing illnesses like HIV and hepatitis C. Antiretroviral treatment (Craftsmanship) addresses a fruitful designated way to deal with repress different phases of the HIV life cycle. Various classes of antiretroviral drugs, including protease inhibitors and integrase inhibitors, target viral catalysts, keeping the infection from repeating and decreasing the viral burden in patients with HIV.

The advancement of direct-acting antivirals (DAAs) has changed the scene of hepatitis C treatment. These designated treatments explicitly repress viral proteins fundamental for the replication of the hepatitis C infection. DAAs offer high fix rates with more limited treatment terms and less secondary effects contrasted with past regimens, making them a foundation in the administration of hepatitis C.

Accuracy medication, directed by designated treatment draws near, has turned into a point of convergence in the treatment of neurodegenerative issues. Alzheimer's illness, described by the amassing of beta-amyloid plaques in the mind, has seen the improvement of designated treatments expecting to change sickness movement.

Monoclonal antibodies like aducanumab have been intended to target and clear beta-amyloid plaques, addressing a clever way to deal with Alzheimer's infection treatment.

In Parkinson's illness, a neurodegenerative issue including the deficiency of dopamine-delivering neurons, designated treatments plan to lighten engine side effects. Profound cerebrum feeling (DBS) is a careful mediation that includes embedding terminals in unambiguous mind locales and regulating their action to mitigate engine side effects related with Parkinson's illness. While not a pharmacological treatment,

DBS epitomizes the designated and customized nature of mediations in neurodegenerative issues.

Regardless of the astounding accomplishments of designated treatments, difficulties and contemplations endure. One critical test is the advancement of opposition after some time. Disease cells, specifically, can develop and adjust, securing changes that render designated treatments less successful. Understanding the systems of opposition and creating techniques to survive or forestall it stay dynamic areas of examination.

Recognizing reasonable atomic focuses for specific sicknesses represents another test. Not all conditions have clear cut atomic targets, making it challenging to foster designated treatments. The heterogeneity of sicknesses, especially in disease, represents a test in recognizing a solitary objective that can really treat all patients with a particular kind of malignant growth.

The expense of designated treatments is an element that raises concerns. These medications frequently include complex assembling processes, adding to their significant expenses. Admittance to designated treatments can be restricted, particularly in districts with monetary requirements or where medical care frameworks might confront hardships in covering the costs related with these high level therapies.

Moral contemplations additionally become possibly the most important factor in the domain of designated treatments, especially with regards to hereditary testing. The data got from hereditary testing brings up issues about protection, assent, and the potential for segregation in view of hereditary inclinations. Finding some kind of harmony between propelling clinical information and safeguarding people's privileges and protection stays a basic thought.

Chapter 4

Immunotherapy Breakthroughs

Immunotherapy, a progressive way to deal with treating different illnesses, has seen surprising forward leaps lately. This creative field outfits the body's safe framework to battle infections, going from disease to immune system issues. The headway made in immunotherapy has opened new roads for treatment, offering desire to patients confronting already unrealistic difficulties.

Quite possibly of the main forward leap in immunotherapy is the advancement of resistant designated spot inhibitors. These inhibitors target explicit proteins on resistant cells, for example, PD-1 and CTLA-4, which go about as brakes on the safe framework. By obstructing these inhibitory signs, safe designated spot inhibitors release the maximum capacity of the insusceptible framework, empowering it to actually perceive and go after disease cells more.

The endorsement of the principal resistant designated spot inhibitor, ipilimumab, denoted a turning point in malignant growth treatment. It showed the way that the resistant framework could be activated to battle malignant growth, prompting strong reactions and further developed endurance rates in patients with cutting edge melanoma. Ensuing improvements in this class of medications, including pembrolizumab and nivolumab, have extended their application to different diseases, including lung, kidney, and bladder malignant growths.

Past invulnerable designated spot inhibitors, another earth shattering immunotherapeutic methodology includes illusory antigen receptor White blood cell treatment, usually known as Vehicle T treatment. This method includes separating a patient's Immune system microorganisms, hereditarily changing them to communicate a receptor intended for malignant growth cells, and afterward mixing the adjusted cells back into the patient. Vehicle T treatment has exhibited noteworthy progress in treating specific blood malignant growths, like leukemia and lymphoma, accomplishing uncommon reaction rates and, surprisingly, prompting total reduction now and again.

The excursion of Vehicle T treatment from exploratory to standard treatment represents the extraordinary force of immunotherapy. The endorsement of the primary Vehicle T treatment, tisagenlecleucel, for the treatment of pediatric intense lymphoblastic leukemia denoted a noteworthy second in the field. Ensuing endorsements, including axicabtagene ciloleucel for particular sorts of lymphoma, highlight the capability of Vehicle T treatment to reclassify the norm of care for explicit diseases.

Notwithstanding malignant growth, immunotherapy has shown guarantee in tending to immune system sicknesses, where the safe framework erroneously goes after sound tissues. Monoclonal antibodies, a sort of immunotherapy, have been created to target explicit particles engaged with the immune system process. For instance, the endorsement of rituximab for rheumatoid joint pain and other immune system conditions features the helpful capability of accuracy immunotherapy in dealing with these mind boggling sicknesses.

The outcome of immunotherapy in assorted clinical fields has provoked scientists to investigate its application in irresistible sicknesses. Immunizations, a customary type of immunotherapy, have been instrumental in forestalling irresistible sicknesses for a really long time. Late advances, like mRNA immunization innovation, have sped up the turn of events and arrangement of antibodies, as shown by the quick making of Coronavirus immunizations.

The mRNA immunizations produced for Coronavirus address a victory of immunotherapy. These immunizations influence the body's own cell hardware to deliver viral proteins, getting a vigorous safe reaction. The speed at which mRNA antibodies were created and their high adequacy in forestalling serious disease and demise have displayed the adaptability and spryness of immunotherapy in answering arising dangers.

While the previously mentioned forward leaps have moved immunotherapy into the spotlight, progressing research keeps on revealing new roads and refine existing methodologies. One area of extraordinary examination includes the distinguishing proof of novel safe designated spots and the advancement of inhibitors focusing on them. This growing scene of safe designated spot regulation holds the commitment of improving the viability of immunotherapy across a more extensive range of malignant growths.

Blends of various immunotherapeutic specialists have arisen as another promising methodology. By utilizing the integral instruments of different therapies, scientists plan to make collaborations that improve the general enemy of malignant growth insusceptible reaction. The idea of mix immunotherapy has previously shown outcome in clinical preliminaries, for certain blends exhibiting better adequacy analyzed than single-specialist treatments.

The microbiome, comprising of trillions of microorganisms dwelling in the human body, has likewise arisen as a basic variable impacting the viability of immunotherapy. Research shows that the piece of the microbiome can influence how the resistant framework answers disease treatment. Controlling the microbiome through probiotics, waste microbiota transplantation, or different mediations presents a clever road for upgrading immunotherapy results.

In the domain of Vehicle T treatment, endeavors are in progress to grow its relevance to strong cancers, which present special difficulties contrasted with blood diseases. Beating impediments like the immunosuppressive growth microenvironment and recognizing appropriate focuses for Vehicle White blood cells on strong cancers are dynamic areas of examination. Outcome in this try could expand the advantages of Vehicle T treatment to a more extensive scope of malignant growth types.

The field of immunotherapy isn't without difficulties and contemplations. Resistant related unfriendly occasions, where the safe framework erroneously goes after typical tissues, can happen with immunotherapy. Finding some kind of harmony between releasing the invulnerable framework's power and forestalling mischief to solid tissues stays a sensitive test. Progressing research plans to refine the comprehension of these occasions and foster systems to alleviate their effect.

One more test lies in understanding and conquering protection from immunotherapy. While certain patients experience sturdy reactions, others show starting advantages followed by backslide. Exploring the elements adding to opposition and creating systems to defeat it are essential for expanding the effect of immunotherapy across a more extensive patient populace.

The monetary contemplations related with immunotherapy additionally warrant consideration. The significant expenses of a few immunotherapeutic specialists, especially Vehicle T treatments, present difficulties to boundless reception.

Endeavors to streamline fabricating processes, diminish creation costs, and investigate elective estimating models are in progress to make these notable treatments more open to a bigger number of patients.

Taking everything into account, the scene of immunotherapy is persistently developing, with forward leaps changing the therapy worldview for malignant growth, immune system illnesses, irresistible infections, and then some. The progress of safe designated spot inhibitors, Vehicle T treatment, mRNA immunizations, and accuracy immunotherapy in different clinical fields features the capability of bridling the resistant framework to stand up to a wide exhibit of wellbeing challenges.

As examination advances, the distinguishing proof of new invulnerable designated spots, the investigation of blend immunotherapies, and the coordination of microbiome contemplations vow to additional upgrade the viability and pertinence of immunotherapy. Difficulties, for example, invulnerable related antagonistic occasions and protection from treatment highlight the intricacy of exploring the sensitive harmony between remedial advantage and expected hurt.

The continuous quest for information and development in immunotherapy holds the commitment of proceeded with forward leaps, offering desire to patients and reshaping the scene of medication. With every headway, immunotherapy draws nearer to understanding its maximum capacity as a groundbreaking power in medical care, giving additional opportunities to patients and clinicians the same.

4.1 Explanation of the immune system's role in fighting cancer

The safe framework, a mind boggling organization of cells, tissues, and organs, assumes a vital part in protecting the body against unsafe trespassers, including disease cells. Understanding the complexities of the resistant framework's reaction to disease is fundamental for valuing the meaning of immunotherapy and other immuno-modulatory approaches in malignant growth treatment.

At its center, the invulnerable framework is intended to recognize the body's own cells (self) and unfamiliar substances (non-self). This capacity to perceive and mount a guard against unfamiliar intruders is coordinated by a different exhibit of invulnerable cells, each with particular capabilities. Two essential parts of the safe framework, the natural resistant framework and the versatile invulnerable framework, work in show to give a complete protection against dangers.

The natural resistant framework fills in as the body's most memorable line of safe-guard. It incorporates actual hindrances like the skin and mucous films, as well as cell parts like neutrophils, macrophages, and normal executioner (NK) cells. These cells are prepared to rapidly recognize and wipe out unfamiliar substances. For instance, macrophages overwhelm and process microorganisms, while NK cells target and obliterate tainted or unusual cells, including malignant growth cells.

The versatile safe framework, then again, gives a more particular and designated re-action. It comprises of Lymphocytes and B cells, which are white platelets that assume vital parts in safe reconnaissance and memory. Lymphocytes are especially significant with regards to disease resistance, as they can perceive and dispose of explicit strange cells, including those changed into destructive states.

One vital instrument by which Lymphocytes distinguish and take out malignant growth cells is through the acknowledgment of antigens. Antigens are atoms that can set off a resistant reaction, and malignant growth cells frequently show interesting antigens that recognize them from ordinary cells. Immune system microorganisms can perceive these disease explicit antigens, empowering them to target and go after malignant growth cells while saving sound tissues specifically.

The interaction by which Lymphocytes perceive and answer disease cells is worked with by significant histocompatibility complex (MHC) atoms. MHC atoms present antigens on the outer layer of cells, permitting Immune system microorganisms to cooperate with and perceive these antigens. The collaboration between Lymphocytes and malignant growth cells is a finely tuned process that includes the acknowledg-ment of explicit antigens and the enactment of invulnerable reactions to kill the strange cells.

Be that as it may, disease cells have developed components to sidestep location and annihilation by the safe framework. One such component includes the outflow of invulnerable designated spot atoms on the outer layer of malignant growth cells.

These designated spot particles, like PD-L1 (modified passing ligand 1), can connect with comparing receptors on Immune system microorganisms, prompting Lymphocyte depletion or inactivation.

The invulnerable designated spot pathway goes about as an administrative instrument to forestall over the top resistant reactions and keep up with insusceptible framework homeostasis. With regards to malignant growth, however, it very well may be taken advantage of by disease cells to get away from safe observation. At the point when PD-L1 on disease cells ties to its receptor, PD-1, on Immune system microorganisms, it conveys inhibitory messages that hose Lymphocyte movement, permitting malignant growth cells to sidestep annihilation.

This avoidance system has prompted the improvement of safe designated spot inhibitors, a class of immunotherapeutic specialists intended to hinder the communication between PD-1 and PD-L1, consequently reactivating Lymphocytes and upgrading their capacity to perceive and kill disease cells. The progress of safe designated spot inhibitors, for example, pembrolizumab and nivolumab, in treating different tumors highlights the significance of defeating resistant avoidance components in malignant growth treatment.

One more basic part of the safe reaction against malignant growth includes the cancer microenvironment. Growths are not homogeneous masses of cells; all things considered, they comprise of a complicated microenvironment that incorporates disease cells, invulnerable cells, veins, and connective tissue. The cooperations inside this microenvironment impact the movement of malignant growth and the adequacy of invulnerable reactions.

Malignant growth cells can control the cancer microenvironment to make an immunosuppressive milieu, upsetting the capacity of resistant cells to mount a compelling reaction. Factors like the arrival of immunosuppressive particles and the enrollment of administrative Lymphocytes (Tregs) add to the foundation of a climate that safeguards malignant growth cells from resistant assault.

Endeavors to upgrade the resistant framework's capacity to penetrate and work inside the growth microenvironment have turned into a focal point of exploration in disease immunotherapy. Systems incorporate consolidating insusceptible designated spot inhibitors with other immunotherapeutic specialists, for example, cytokines or agonists that invigorate invulnerable cell action. By tweaking the growth microenvironment, specialists intend to make conditions that favor a vigorous and supported safe reaction against disease.

Notwithstanding Lymphocytes, one more central participant in the versatile safe framework is B cells. B cells produce antibodies, which are proteins that can perceive and tie to explicit antigens. While antibodies are generally connected with irresistible illnesses, they likewise assume a part in disease resistance. Antibodies can target malignant growth cells straightforwardly or can be utilized as vehicles for conveying helpful specialists to disease cells.

Monoclonal antibodies, a class of immunotherapeutic specialists, are intended to copy the safe framework's capacity to deliver antibodies. These antibodies can be designed to straightforwardly perceive explicit antigens on the outer layer of malignant growth cells, empowering them to target and kill disease cells. Rituximab, for instance, is a monoclonal immunizer utilized in the treatment of particular kinds of lymphoma by focusing on CD20, a particle communicated on the outer layer of B cells.

The connection between the insusceptible framework and disease is a dynamic and diverse interaction. The advancing comprehension of this association has prompted the improvement of different immunotherapeutic techniques pointed toward saddling the safe framework's ability to battle disease. Past safe designated spot inhibitors and monoclonal antibodies, receptive cell treatments, like Vehicle T treatment, address a progressive methodology in which a patient's own resistant cells are designed to target and dispose of malignant growth.

Vehicle T treatment includes the extraction of Immune system microorganisms from a patient, hereditary change to communicate an illusory antigen receptor (Vehicle) well defined for disease cells, and reinfusion of the adjusted cells into the patient.

This customized and designated approach has exhibited surprising achievement, especially in the therapy of specific blood malignant growths, where Vehicle Lymphocytes have shown the capacity to prompt strong reductions and, at times, a fix.

The progress of immunotherapy in treating disease has prodded continuous examination to grow its application to a more extensive scope of disease types and work on its viability. Mix treatments, which include the utilization of different immunotherapeutic specialists with corresponding components of activity, have shown guarantee in clinical preliminaries. By tending to various parts of the safe reaction and beating potential obstruction systems, blend approaches look to improve the general viability of immunotherapy.

The job of the resistant framework in battling disease reaches out past the direct focusing of malignant growth cells. The idea of malignant growth immunosurveillance, proposed by Dr. Robert Schreiber, proposes that the insusceptible framework effectively screens and kills arising disease cells before they can form into clinically perceptible growths. This continuous reconnaissance features the powerful exchange between the invulnerable framework and the advancing scene of disease advancement.

While the resistant framework has amazing capacities, disease cells can in any case take advantage of different components to dodge recognition and disposal. Research endeavors are coordinated toward understanding and conquering these avoidance systems. The field of malignant growth immunotherapy keeps on advancing quickly, with continuous clinical preliminaries investigating novel specialists, blend draws near, and inventive advancements to improve the safe framework's capacity to perceive and kill disease.

The progress of immunotherapy in malignant growth treatment epitomizes the extraordinary capability of outfitting the body's own guards. From resistant designated spot inhibitors that discharge the brakes on Lymphocytes to Vehicle T treatment that engineers safe cells for accuracy focusing on, these headways highlight the flexibility and versatility of the insusceptible framework in the battle against malignant growth.

All in all, the resistant framework's job in battling malignant growth is a dynamic and unpredictable cycle including numerous parts and connections. From the underlying acknowledgment of malignant growth explicit antigens to the intricate transaction inside the cancer microenvironment, the safe reaction against disease is a finely tuned organization. Immunotherapy, through different modalities, exploits and upgrades these regular guard instruments to give new roads to malignant growth treatment, offering desire to patients and reshaping the scene of oncology. As our comprehension develops, the excursion of immunotherapy proceeds, set apart by leap forwards that reclassify conceivable outcomes and enlighten the way toward more compelling and customized disease treatments.

4.2 Overview of recent breakthroughs in immunotherapy

As of late, immunotherapy has arisen as a groundbreaking power in the field of medication, offering creative ways to deal with treating different illnesses, with disease at the very front. Leap forwards in immunotherapy have reshaped treatment ideal models, giving new expectation and further developed results for patients. This outline investigates key ongoing forward leaps in immunotherapy, spreading over advancements in resistant designated spot inhibitors, Vehicle T treatment, oncolytic infections, and customized antibodies.

Invulnerable designated spot inhibitors address a noteworthy class of immunotherapeutic specialists that have changed malignant growth treatment. These inhibitors target explicit proteins on invulnerable cells, like PD-1 (customized cell demise protein 1) and CTLA-4 (cytotoxic T-lymphocyte-related protein 4), which go about as administrative brakes on the insusceptible framework. By obstructing these inhibitory signs, resistant designated spot inhibitors release the maximum capacity of Lymphocytes, empowering them to successfully perceive and go after malignant growth cells more.

The endorsement of ipilimumab in 2011 denoted a noteworthy achievement as the main safe designated spot inhibitor for disease treatment. Ipilimumab targets CTLA-4 and exhibited huge upgrades in generally endurance for patients with cutting edge melanoma. Resulting endorsements of PD-1 inhibitors, for example, pembrolizumab and nivolumab, extended the utilization of invulnerable designated spot inhibitors to different disease types, including lung, kidney, and bladder tumors.

One striking part of resistant designated spot inhibitors is their capacity to prompt sturdy reactions in a subset of patients. A few people experience delayed times of infectious prevention, recommending the foundation of insusceptible memory against disease. The sturdiness of reactions has tested conventional ideas of malignant growth as an unyielding and moderate sickness, offering the possibility of long haul control and expected fixes.

Mix systems have additionally progressed the field of insusceptible designated spot hindrance. The utilization of double designated spot barricade, focusing on both PD-1 and CTLA-4 all the while, has shown upgraded adequacy in specific malignant growths. For instance, the blend of nivolumab and ipilimumab has been endorsed for the treatment of cutting edge melanoma, showing better results thought about than monotherapy.

Past resistant designated spot inhibitors, illusory antigen receptor White blood cell treatment (Vehicle T treatment) addresses a progressive methodology in malignant growth treatment. Vehicle T treatment includes the extraction of a patient's Immune system microorganisms, hereditary change to communicate a receptor intended for malignant growth cells, and reinfusion of the adjusted cells back into the patient. This customized and designated technique has shown exceptional progress in treating specific hematological malignancies.

The endorsement of the principal Vehicle T treatment, tisagenlecleucel, for pediatric intense lymphoblastic leukemia denoted a notable second in the field. Resulting endorsements, including axicabtagene ciloleucel for particular kinds of lymphoma, highlight the capability of Vehicle T treatment to reclassify the norm of care for explicit malignant growths. Vehicle T treatment has accomplished noteworthy reaction rates, including total abatements, in patients who had depleted regular treatment choices.

Notwithstanding, challenges continue expanding the progress of Vehicle T treatment to strong growths. Strong growths present a more mind boggling microenvironment, with hindrances, for example, immunosuppression and actual boundaries restricting the invasion and capability of Vehicle White blood cells. Continuous investigation plans to conquer these difficulties, investigating procedures to improve Vehicle Immune system microorganism diligence and viability in strong cancer settings.

Oncolytic infections address one more encouraging road in immunotherapy. These infections are designed to taint and obliterate disease cells while saving ordinary cells specifically. Notwithstanding their direct oncolytic impacts, these infections invigorate against cancer invulnerable reactions by delivering growth related antigens and advancing the enactment of resistant cells inside the growth microenvironment.

Talimogene laherparepvec (T-VEC), an oncolytic herpes simplex infection, was the first oncolytic infection to get FDA endorsement for the treatment of cutting edge melanoma. T-VEC exhibited a double component of activity by straightforwardly lysing malignant growth cells and inciting foundational hostile to cancer insusceptible reactions. The outcome of T-VEC has prodded continuous investigation into the advancement of oncolytic infections for different malignant growth types.

In the domain of customized medication, disease immunizations custom-made to a singular's particular growth antigens definitely stand out enough to be noticed. These immunizations mean to animate the safe framework to perceive and go after disease cells bearing patient-explicit transformations. Neoantigens, which emerge from growth explicit transformations, act as ideal focuses for customized disease antibodies.

Ongoing forward leaps in cutting edge sequencing and bioinformatics have worked with the ID of neoantigens with high accuracy. This information empowers the plan of customized immunizations that trigger safe reactions against the remarkable changes present in a singular's cancer. While customized malignant growth antibodies are still in beginning phases of improvement, they hold extraordinary commitment for upgrading the explicitness and adequacy of immunotherapy.

Notwithstanding these significant leap forwards, propels in how we might interpret the microbiome's part in balancing safe reactions have opened new roads for examination and helpful mediations. The structure of the stomach microbiome has been connected to reaction rates to safe designated spot inhibitors, affecting the adequacy of these treatments. Methodologies, for example, waste microbiota transplantation and probiotic mediations are being investigated to improve the stomach microbiome and upgrade immunotherapy results.

The outcome of immunotherapy reaches out past malignant growth, with applications in the treatment of immune system illnesses. Monoclonal antibodies focusing on unambiguous safe cells or particles engaged with immune system processes have exhibited adequacy in conditions like rheumatoid joint pain, psoriasis, and provocative entrail illnesses. These immunomodulatory specialists offer more designated and exact ways to deal with overseeing immune system issues, limiting foundational incidental effects.

As the field of immunotherapy keeps on advancing, scientists are investigating novel targets and remedial modalities. The recognizable proof of extra insusceptible designated spots past PD-1 and CTLA-4 has prompted the improvement of inhibitors focusing on elective pathways. For example, inhibitors of TIM-3, Slack 3, and TIGIT are going through clinical assessment, determined to extend the collection of immunotherapeutic choices.

The idea of mix immunotherapy, including the concurrent or successive utilization of numerous immunotherapeutic specialists, has gotten momentum. By utilizing the integral components of various medicines, analysts mean to improve the general enemy of growth insusceptible reaction. Clinical preliminaries researching different blend techniques, incorporating resistant designated spot inhibitors with designated treatments or different immunotherapies, are in progress across various malignant growth types.

Regardless of the wonderful advancement, challenges persevere in the more extensive reception of immunotherapy. Safe related unfriendly occasions, coming about because of the enactment of the invulnerable framework against ordinary tissues, can happen and require cautious administration. Biomarkers anticipating reaction to immunotherapy are effectively looked to direct treatment choices and recognize patients who are probably going to benefit.

The significant expense of a few immunotherapeutic specialists, especially Vehicle T treatments, presents monetary difficulties and brings up issues about openness.

Endeavors to upgrade fabricating processes, decrease creation costs, and investigate elective valuing models are fundamental to guarantee the more extensive accessibility of these momentous treatments.

All in all, ongoing forward leaps in immunotherapy have changed the scene of disease treatment and then some. From the outcome of safe designated spot inhibitors and Vehicle T treatment to the commitment of oncolytic infections and customized disease immunizations, these developments offer new expectation and opportunities for patients.

The unique interchange between the resistant framework and malignant growth keeps on being a point of convergence of exploration, driving the improvement of novel immunotherapeutic techniques and propelling the field toward additional compelling and customized medicines. As the excursion of immunotherapy unfurls, the cooperative endeavors of specialists, clinicians, and industry accomplices hold the way to opening further leap forwards and further developing results for patients confronting complex clinical difficulties.

4.3 Successful immunotherapy treatments

Immunotherapy, a progressive way to deal with treating illnesses, has exhibited striking outcome in different clinical fields, especially in the therapy of disease and immune system problems. Fruitful immunotherapy medicines have reshaped the scene of medication, offering new desire to patients confronting beforehand testing and frequently desperate determinations. This outline investigates key instances of effective immunotherapy medicines, featuring leap forwards in resistant designated spot inhibitors, Vehicle T treatment, oncolytic infections, and accuracy immunotherapy.

Invulnerable designated spot inhibitors, a class of immunotherapeutic specialists, have arisen as exceptionally effective therapies for different diseases. These inhibitors target explicit proteins on invulnerable cells, like PD-1 (customized cell passing protein 1) and CTLA-4 (cytotoxic T-lymphocyte-related protein 4), which go about as brakes on the resistant framework. By impeding these inhibitory signs, resistant designated spot inhibitors release the maximum capacity of Immune system microorganisms, empowering them to actually perceive and go after malignant growth cells more.

One of the spearheading examples of overcoming adversity in safe designated spot hindrance is the endorsement of ipilimumab for the treatment of cutting edge melanoma. Ipilimumab targets CTLA-4 and has exhibited huge upgrades in by and large endurance for patients with metastatic melanoma, a generally moving malignant growth to treat. This achievement prepared for the turn of events and endorsement of PD-1 inhibitors, including pembrolizumab and nivolumab, which extended the utilization of insusceptible designated spot inhibitors to different disease types.

One of the surprising parts of safe designated spot inhibitors is their capacity to prompt strong reactions in a subset of patients. A few people experience long haul control of their sickness, testing regular thoughts of disease as an unyielding and moderate condition. For instance, patients with metastatic melanoma treated with pembrolizumab or nivolumab have shown supported reactions, with an eminent extent encountering tough complete reductions.

Blend systems have additionally upgraded the progress of resistant designated spot restraint. The mix of nivolumab and ipilimumab, which targets both PD-1 and CTLA-4 at the same time, has shown better viability thought about than monotherapy in specific tumors, like high level melanoma. The synergistic impacts of double designated spot bar highlight the potential for combinatorial ways to deal with amplify restorative advantage.

Fanciful Antigen Receptor White blood cell treatment (Vehicle T treatment) addresses one more forward leap in disease treatment, especially for specific hematological malignancies. Vehicle T treatment includes the extraction of a patient's Lymphocytes, hereditary change to communicate a fanciful antigen receptor (Vehicle) well defined for disease cells, and reinfusion of the changed cells back into the patient. This customized and designated approach has exhibited remarkable outcome in clinical preliminaries.

The endorsement of tisagenlecleucel for pediatric intense lymphoblastic leukemia denoted a memorable second in the field of Vehicle T treatment. Kids with backslid or unmanageable leukemia who got tisagenlecleucel accomplished astounding reaction rates, with some encountering total abatements. Ensuing endorsements, including axicabtagene ciloleucel for particular kinds of lymphoma, highlight the capability of Vehicle T treatment to rethink the norm of care for explicit malignant growths.

Vehicle T treatment's prosperity isn't restricted to pediatric leukemia; it has shown guarantee in treating grown-up patients with forceful lymphomas. Patients who have depleted regular treatment choices, including chemotherapy and undeveloped cell transplantation, have accomplished sturdy reactions with Vehicle T treatment. The capacity of Vehicle Lymphocytes to continue in the body and keep up with their enemy of cancer action over a drawn out period is a vital consider the treatment's prosperity.

While Vehicle T treatment has exhibited striking outcome in hematological malignancies, stretching out its viability to strong cancers presents difficulties. Strong growths present a more perplexing microenvironment, portrayed by immunosuppression and actual hindrances that limit the invasion and capability of Vehicle White blood cells. Conquering these difficulties is a functioning area of exploration, with continuous endeavors to improve Vehicle Lymphocyte steadiness and viability in strong cancer settings.

Oncolytic infections address one more road of fruitful immunotherapy, with the possibility to treat different diseases. These infections are designed to contaminate and annihilate disease cells while saving typical cells specifically. The oncolytic cycle straightforwardly kills disease cells as well as animates hostile to cancer safe reactions by delivering growth related antigens and advancing the actuation of resistant cells inside the cancer microenvironment.

Talimogene laherparepvec (T-VEC), an oncolytic herpes simplex infection, got FDA endorsement for the treatment of cutting edge melanoma. T-VEC's prosperity lies in its double component of activity — straightforwardly lysing disease cells and actuating fundamental enemy of cancer resistant reactions. The endorsement of T-VEC denoted a huge achievement in the improvement of oncolytic infections as a feasible and viable remedial choice for disease patients.

The outcome of T-VEC has prodded continuous examination into the advancement of oncolytic infections for different disease types. Rigvir, an oncolytic infection got from the Reverberation 7 intestinal infection, has shown guarantee in the treatment of melanoma. Clinical preliminaries examining oncolytic infections, including those designed to target explicit disease types, keep on propelling, offering additional opportunities for patients with a scope of malignancies.

Accuracy immunotherapy, including the recognizable proof and focusing of explicit particles or pathways engaged with the safe reaction, has additionally added to effective treatment results. Monoclonal antibodies, a type of accuracy immunotherapy, have been created to target explicit particles on safe cells or disease cells. Rituximab, for instance, targets CD20 on B cells and is utilized in the treatment of particular kinds of lymphoma and immune system sicknesses.

Customized disease immunizations, custom-made to a singular's particular growth antigens, address one more part of accuracy immunotherapy. These immunizations intend to invigorate the invulnerable framework to perceive and go after malignant growth cells bearing patient-explicit transformations. Propels in cutting edge sequencing and bioinformatics have worked with the ID of neoantigens, which emerge from growth explicit transformations and act as ideal focuses for customized disease antibodies.

While customized disease immunizations are still in beginning phases of improvement, they hold extraordinary commitment for upgrading the particularity and viability of immunotherapy. The idea of preparing the resistant framework to perceive and focus on the exceptional transformations present in a singular's growth mirrors the rising pattern toward customized and accuracy medication in disease treatment.

Past malignant growth, immunotherapy has shown outcome in the treatment of immune system sicknesses. Monoclonal antibodies focusing on unambiguous safe cells or atoms engaged with immune system processes have shown viability in conditions like rheumatoid joint pain, psoriasis, and provocative gut sicknesses. These immunomodulatory specialists offer designated and exact ways to deal with overseeing immune system issues, limiting foundational secondary effects.

The progress of immunotherapy medicines reaches out past the singular modalities to the aggregate effect of mix systems. Combinatorial methodologies including different immunotherapeutic specialists, like safe designated spot inhibitors with designated treatments or different immunotherapies, have shown guarantee in clinical preliminaries. By tending to different parts of the invulnerable reaction and defeating potential obstruction systems, mix immunotherapy looks to upgrade the general viability of treatment.

Regardless of these victories, difficulties and contemplations persevere in the more extensive reception of immunotherapy. Invulnerable related unfriendly occasions, coming about because of the actuation of the insusceptible framework against ordinary tissues, can happen and require cautious administration. Biomarkers anticipating reaction to immunotherapy are effectively tried to direct treatment choices and distinguish patients who are probably going to benefit.

The monetary contemplations related for certain immunotherapeutic specialists, especially Vehicle T treatments, likewise warrant consideration. The significant expenses of these momentous treatments present difficulties to inescapable reception. Endeavors to enhance fabricating processes, lessen creation costs, and investigate elective evaluating models are fundamental for make these medicines more open to a bigger number of patients.

Immunotherapy, a progressive way to deal with treating sicknesses by outfitting the body's own safe framework, has seen extraordinary outcome as of late. From the therapy of disease to immune system problems, immunotherapy has arisen as an extraordinary power in medication, offering new expectation and further developed results for patients confronting different wellbeing challenges. This extensive outline investigates key immunotherapy therapies, including invulnerable designated spot inhibitors, fanciful antigen receptor Lymphocyte treatment (Vehicle T treatment), oncolytic infections, monoclonal antibodies, and customized malignant growth immunizations.

Invulnerable Designated spot Inhibitors:

Safe designated spot inhibitors have arisen as a foundation of fruitful immunotherapy, especially in the field of malignant growth treatment. These inhibitors target explicit proteins on resistant cells, for example, PD-1 and CTLA-4, which go about as administrative brakes on the safe framework. By obstructing these inhibitory signs, invulnerable designated spot inhibitors release the maximum capacity of Lymphocytes, empowering them to actually perceive and go after malignant growth cells more.

The endorsement of ipilimumab, a resistant designated spot inhibitor focusing on CTLA-4, denoted a turning point in disease treatment. Ipilimumab showed huge enhancements in by and large endurance for patients with cutting edge melanoma, a generally moving malignant growth to treat. Resulting improvements in PD-1 inhibitors, including pembrolizumab and nivolumab, extended the utilization of resistant designated spot inhibitors to different disease types, including lung, kidney, and bladder malignant growths.

One noteworthy part of safe designated spot inhibitors is their capacity to prompt sturdy reactions in a subset of patients. A few people experience delayed times of infectious prevention, testing customary thoughts of malignant growth as an inflexible and moderate sickness. Eminently, patients with metastatic melanoma treated with

PD-1 inhibitors have exhibited supported reactions, with a critical extent encountering tough complete reductions.

Blend techniques have additionally improved the progress of safe designated spot hindrance. The blend of nivolumab and ipilimumab, focusing on both PD-1 and CTLA-4 at the same time, has shown better adequacy analyzed than monotherapy in specific malignant growths, like high level melanoma. The synergistic impacts of double designated spot bar highlight the potential for combinatorial ways to deal with amplify helpful advantage.

Vehicle T Treatment:

Illusory Antigen Receptor Immune system microorganism treatment, or Vehicle T treatment, addresses a weighty methodology in disease treatment, especially for specific hematological malignancies. This customized and designated treatment includes separating a patient's Immune system microorganisms, hereditarily changing them to communicate an illusory antigen receptor (Vehicle) well defined for malignant growth cells, and reinfusing the adjusted cells back into the patient.

The endorsement of tisagenlecleucel for pediatric intense lymphoblastic leukemia denoted a noteworthy accomplishment in Vehicle T treatment. Kids with backslid or hard-headed leukemia treated with tisagenlecleucel accomplished wonderful reaction rates, with some encountering total reductions. Ensuing endorsements, including axicabtagene ciloleucel for particular kinds of lymphoma, highlight the capability of Vehicle T treatment to rethink the norm of care for explicit diseases.

The outcome of Vehicle T treatment reaches out past pediatric leukemia to grown-up patients with forceful lymphomas. Patients who have depleted customary treatment choices, including chemotherapy and immature microorganism transplantation, have accomplished solid reactions with Vehicle T treatment. The capacity of Vehicle Lymphocytes to endure in the body and keep up with their enemy of growth action over a lengthy period is a critical figure the treatment's prosperity.

Notwithstanding, challenges continue broadening the progress of Vehicle T treatment to strong cancers. Strong growths present a more perplexing microenvironment, portrayed by immunosuppression and actual hindrances that limit the invasion and capability of Vehicle White blood cells. Continuous exploration is centered around defeating these difficulties, with endeavors to upgrade Vehicle Lymphocyte diligence and adequacy in strong growth settings.

Oncolytic Infections:

Oncolytic infections address one more encouraging road in fruitful immunotherapy. These infections are designed to taint and obliterate malignant growth cells while saving typical cells specifically. The oncolytic interaction straightforwardly kills malignant growth cells as well as invigorates hostile to cancer invulnerable reactions by delivering growth related antigens and advancing the actuation of safe cells inside the cancer microenvironment.

Talimogene laherparepvec (T-VEC), an oncolytic herpes simplex infection, got FDA endorsement for the treatment of cutting edge melanoma. T-VEC's prosperity lies in its double component of activity — straightforwardly lysing disease cells and prompting fundamental enemy of cancer resistant reactions. The endorsement of T-VEC denoted a huge achievement in the improvement of oncolytic infections as a reasonable and powerful remedial choice for disease patients.

The progress of T-VEC has prodded continuous examination into the improvement of oncolytic infections for different malignant growth types. Rigvir, an oncolytic infection got from the Reverberation 7 intestinal infection, has shown guarantee in the treatment of melanoma. Clinical preliminaries examining oncolytic infections, including those designed to target explicit disease types, keep on propelling, offering additional opportunities for patients with a scope of malignancies.

Monoclonal Antibodies:

Monoclonal antibodies, a type of accuracy immunotherapy, play had an essential impact in effective therapies for malignant growth and immune system illnesses. These antibodies are intended to target explicit atoms on safe cells or disease cells, balancing resistant reactions and adding to remedial viability.

Rituximab, a monoclonal neutralizer focusing on CD20 on B cells, has shown progress in the treatment of particular kinds of lymphoma and immune system illnesses like rheumatoid joint pain. The designated approach of monoclonal antibodies limits blow-back to typical tissues, bringing about additional particular and very much endured treatments.

Customized Disease Immunizations:

Customized disease immunizations address a state of the art boondocks in immunotherapy. These immunizations are custom fitted to a singular's particular growth antigens, intending to invigorate the invulnerable framework to perceive and go after disease cells bearing patient-explicit changes. Propels in cutting edge sequencing and bioinformatics have worked with the distinguishing proof of neoantigens, which emerge from growth explicit transformations and act as ideal focuses for customized disease antibodies.

While customized disease immunizations are still in beginning phases of advancement, they hold extraordinary commitment for improving the particularity and adequacy of immunotherapy. The idea of preparing the resistant framework to perceive and focus on the novel changes present in a singular's growth mirrors the rising pattern toward customized and accuracy medication in disease treatment.

Victories Past Disease:

Immunotherapy victories stretch out past malignant growth to the treatment of immune system infections. Monoclonal antibodies focusing on unambiguous resistant cells or atoms engaged with immune system processes have shown adequacy in conditions like rheumatoid joint pain, psoriasis, and provocative gut illnesses. These immunomodulatory specialists offer designated and exact ways to deal with overseeing immune system problems, limiting foundational aftereffects.

Difficulties and Contemplations:

Regardless of these victories, difficulties and contemplations endure in the more extensive reception of immunotherapy. Safe related antagonistic occasions, coming about because of the initiation of the resistant framework against ordinary tissues, can happen and require cautious administration. Biomarkers anticipating reaction to immunotherapy are effectively tried to direct treatment choices and recognize patients who are probably going to benefit.

The monetary contemplations related for certain immunotherapeutic specialists, especially Vehicle T treatments, additionally warrant consideration. The significant expenses of these notable treatments present difficulties to far reaching reception. Endeavors to upgrade fabricating processes, diminish creation costs, and investigate elective evaluating models are fundamental for make these medicines more open to a bigger number of patients.

Chapter 5

Gene Editing and CRISPR Technology

Quality altering and CRISPR (Grouped Consistently Interspaced Short Palindromic Rehashes) innovation have arisen as progressive devices in the field of hereditary qualities, offering uncommon capacities to control the hereditary code of living life forms. This mechanical advancement has opened new roads for treating hereditary problems, grasping major natural cycles, and in any event, designing advantageous characteristics in different living beings.

At the core of quality altering lies the CRISPR-Cas9 framework, a sub-atomic instrument that permits exact change of DNA groupings. The framework is gotten from the regular safeguard components of microbes and archaea against infections and other unfamiliar bodies. The CRISPR cluster comprises of short, to some extent palindromic rehashed DNA successions, mixed with extraordinary DNA arrangements known as spacers, got from past openings to viral DNA. These spacers act as a memory of past contaminations, permitting the living being to perceive and guard against explicit infections.

The Cas9 protein, an endonuclease chemical, assumes a focal part in the CRISPR framework. It behaves like a couple of "sub-atomic scissors," directed by RNA particles that are integral to the objective DNA succession. At the point when the RNA particle finds its objective DNA arrangement, Cas9 cuts the DNA at that exact area. This cut can then be fixed by the cell's normal fix apparatus, acquainting changes with the hereditary code simultaneously.

One of the vital benefits of CRISPR innovation is its capacity to be modified for explicit quality altering assignments. Scientists can plan engineered RNA atoms that match the objective DNA arrangement, taking into account exact and coordinated adjustments. This degree of control has reformed hereditary designing, making it more open and proficient than any time in recent memory.

The likely utilizations of quality altering and CRISPR innovation are immense and shifted. One of the most encouraging regions is the treatment of hereditary problems.

Acquired illnesses brought about by changes in a solitary quality might possibly be remedied utilizing CRISPR innovation. By presenting the right hereditary grouping or fixing the defective one, analysts intend to dispense with or alleviate the impacts of these problems at the hereditary level.

For instance, sicknesses like sickle cell pallor, brought about by a transformation in the HBB quality, are prime contender for CRISPR-based therapies. The capacity to exactly alter the transformed quality and reestablish its generally expected capability holds the commitment of relieving people impacted by such hereditary issues. Clinical preliminaries and progressing research in this space are making ready for the advancement of novel remedial methodologies.

Past treating hereditary sicknesses, CRISPR innovation is likewise being investigated for applications in farming. The capacity to alter the genomes of harvests offers the possibility to upgrade their protection from sicknesses, work on nourishing substance, and increment yields. Scientists are dealing with creating crops that are stronger to natural pressure, like dry season or outrageous temperatures, at last adding to worldwide food security.

Additionally, the change of animals genomes utilizing CRISPR innovation can possibly work on creature wellbeing and upgrade horticultural efficiency. Hereditary adjustments can be acquainted with make creatures more impervious to sicknesses or to upgrade positive characteristics, like meat quality or milk creation. Nonetheless, moral contemplations and public discernments encompassing hereditarily changed organic entities (GMOs) in horticulture stay significant elements to address.

In the domain of medication, CRISPR has additionally opened new roads for disease examination and treatment. The innovation can be utilized to target and adjust explicit qualities related with malignant growth, taking into account more exact and customized treatments.

Also, CRISPR has been utilized in the advancement of creature models for concentrating on different illnesses, giving significant experiences into the hidden systems and likely restorative mediations.

Regardless of its enormous potential, the utilization of CRISPR innovation raises moral worries and prompts conversations about the mindful and moral use of quality altering. The capacity to change the human germline — adjusting the hereditary material that can be given to people in the future — presents huge moral issues. The potential for unseen side-effects and the production of creator infants with upgraded physical or mental capacities bring up issues about the moral and cultural ramifications of such mediations.

The worldwide academic local area perceives the significance of laying out moral rules and guidelines to administer the utilization of CRISPR innovation. Gatherings and meetings have been coordinated to work with conversations among researchers, ethicists, policymakers, and the overall population. Finding some kind of harmony between the possible advantages of quality altering and the moral contemplations encompassing its utilization is pivotal for mindful advancement in this field.

The openness of CRISPR innovation has additionally raised worries about the chance of its abuse. The straightforwardness and moderateness of the innovation make it all the more broadly accessible, expanding the gamble of unapproved and possibly hurtful use. The chance of "biohackers" endeavoring quality altering beyond customary exploration and clinical settings brings up issues about the requirement for severe guidelines and oversight to forestall potentially negative side-effects.

In 2018, Chinese researcher Dr. He Jiankui professed to have made the world's most memorable hereditarily altered children utilizing CRISPR innovation. This declaration started worldwide discussion and judgment, featuring the requirement for clear rules and global joint effort to direct the utilization of quality altering in people. The occurrence highlighted the significance of moral contemplations and the possible outcomes of unregulated quality altering rehearses.

Mainstream researchers answered the contention by stressing the significance of mindful exploration and the requirement for straightforwardness in the turn of events and utilization of quality altering advancements. Requires a ban on germline altering and the foundation of global rules picked up speed, prompting restored conversations on the moral limits of quality altering.

Past the moral contemplations, there are additionally specialized difficulties related with CRISPR innovation. Off-target impacts, where the Cas9 protein inadvertently alters DNA successions other than the expected objective, have been a worry. Specialists are effectively attempting to upgrade the accuracy of CRISPR innovation, limiting askew impacts to guarantee the security and exactness of quality altering applications.

The advancement of option CRISPR frameworks, like CRISPR-Cas12 and CRISPR-Cas13, extends the tool compartment of quality altering methods. These frameworks offer remarkable benefits, including different objective successions and the capacity to alter RNA instead of DNA. Investigating these elective frameworks furnishes specialists with extra choices for explicit applications and addresses a portion of the restrictions related with the first CRISPR-Cas9 framework.

As the field of quality altering keeps on propelling, the moral, legitimate, and social ramifications of this innovation become progressively mind boggling. Worldwide coordinated effort and open exchange are vital for address these difficulties and foster a structure that guarantees the capable and moral utilization of quality altering devices. The Asilomar Meeting on Recombinant DNA in 1975 fills in as a verifiable point of reference, where researchers accumulated to examine the expected dangers and advantages of recombinant DNA innovation, prompting the foundation of rules for its protected use.

The potential for CRISPR innovation to be utilized in improving human abilities or making fashioner children brings up significant moral issues. The idea of "planner children" includes choosing or adjusting explicit characteristics in undeveloped organisms, like knowledge, actual appearance, or even character attributes. This raises worries about the potential for making a general public with expanded social disparity, where people with admittance to quality altering innovations might possess the ability to upgrade their kids' credits.

The possibility of hereditary improvement likewise prompts conversations about the meaning of business as usual and the expected effect on variety inside the human populace. Moral contemplations stretch out past the specialized parts of quality altering to incorporate more extensive cultural ramifications, requiring a smart and comprehensive way to deal with direction.

In the domain of preservation science, CRISPR innovation offers possible answers for address difficulties connected with biodiversity and biological system wellbeing. Endeavors are in progress to investigate the utilization of quality altering to resuscitate wiped out species or upgrade the strength of jeopardized ones. The capacity to adjust the genomes of organic entities to make them more versatile to changing conditions holds guarantee for preservation endeavors notwithstanding environmental change and natural surroundings misfortune.

Be that as it may, the utilization of quality altering in protection likewise raises moral and environmental worries. Bringing hereditarily altered creatures into normal biological systems could have unanticipated results, upsetting existing natural adjusts and cooperations. The potential for accidental mischief to environments and the moral ramifications of modifying the hereditary cosmetics of species in the wild require cautious thought and thorough assessment prior to executing quality altering techniques in preservation rehearses.

In the lawful space, the quick advancement in quality altering has dominated the improvement of far reaching administrative structures. The current administrative scene fluctuates across nations, prompting an absence of normalized rules for the moral and mindful utilization of CRISPR innovation. Global joint effort is fundamental to lay out an orchestrated administrative structure that considers the different moral, social, and cultural viewpoints encompassing quality altering.

The ramifications of quality altering reach out past the research center and into the domains of protection and security. The capacity to control the hereditary code raises worries about the likely abuse of hereditary data, including unapproved admittance to people's hereditary information and the potential for hereditary separation. Shielding hereditary protection and guaranteeing the safe treatment of hereditary data are basic angles that require consideration as quality altering advances become more common.

In the field of irresistible sicknesses, CRISPR innovation has been investigated for its possible in creating novel antiviral procedures. Scientists are exploring the utilization of CRISPR to target and debilitate viral genomes, offering another way to deal with battle viral diseases. The flexibility of CRISPR innovation considers the fast improvement of designated antiviral treatments, giving an expected device in the continuous fight against arising viral dangers.

The crossing point of CRISPR innovation and man-made brainpower (artificial intelligence) holds guarantee for speeding up research and improving the proficiency of quality altering processes. Man-made intelligence calculations can investigate immense datasets, anticipate potential off-target impacts, and upgrade CRISPR plans, smoothing out the exploratory work process. The cooperative energy among man-made intelligence and CRISPR innovation embodies the interdisciplinary idea of current logical exploration and driving development across assorted fields potential.

While the moral conversations encompassing quality altering basically center around its applications in people and creatures, the utilization of CRISPR innovation in microorganisms raises its own arrangement of contemplations. The potential for quality altering to be applied in the alteration of microbes and different microorganisms for modern or ecological purposes presents the two amazing open doors and difficulties.

In the modern area, quality altering can be utilized to improve the development of biofuels, proteins, and other important bioproducts. Designed microorganisms with advanced metabolic pathways can add to additional reasonable and effective modern cycles. Be that as it may, the arrival of hereditarily changed microorganisms into the climate raises natural worries and requires cautious gamble evaluation.

Ecological uses of quality altering reach out to the field of manufactured science, where microorganisms are intended to carry out unambiguous roles, like natural remediation or the evacuation of poisons.

5.1 Introduction to gene editing and CRISPR technology

Quality altering and CRISPR (Bunched Consistently Interspaced Short Palindromic Rehashes) innovation have arisen as extraordinary powers in the domain of atomic science, offering phenomenal accuracy and command over the control of hereditary material. These notable devices have re-imagined the conceivable outcomes of hereditary designing, permitting researchers to alter DNA with unmatched precision and effectiveness.

At the center of this progressive innovation is the CRISPR-Cas9 framework, a sub-atomic device got from the regular guard instruments of microorganisms and archaea against viral contaminations. The CRISPR exhibit comprises of short, somewhat palindromic rehashed DNA arrangements blended with exceptional DNA successions known as spacers, procured from past experiences with infections. This fills in as a memory bank, empowering the living being to perceive and mount protections against explicit viral dangers.

The central member in the CRISPR-Cas9 framework is the Cas9 protein, an endonuclease chemical that goes about as a couple of "sub-atomic scissors." Directed by RNA particles that are intended to be corresponding to the objective DNA grouping, Cas9 definitively cuts the DNA at the expected area. The phone's regular fix systems then, at that point, kick in to fix the cut, permitting analysts to acquaint changes with the hereditary code during the maintenance cycle.

One of the distinctive elements of CRISPR innovation is its programmability. Researchers can plan engineered RNA particles that match the objective DNA grouping, giving a degree of accuracy and customization beforehand inconceivable. This programmability has opened up a bunch of uses, going from remedying hereditary imperfections and getting infections changing yields for expanded versatility and efficiency.

The expected uses of quality altering and CRISPR innovation are broad and significant. One of the essential areas of center is the treatment of hereditary problems. By exactly altering the DNA to address changes liable for sicknesses, scientists expect to foster designated treatments that address the underlying driver of hereditary illnesses. This holds the commitment of changing the scene of medication, offering desire to people with acquired conditions.

Take, for example, the expected use of CRISPR innovation in treating sickle cell weakness — a hereditary problem brought about by a change in the HBB quality. The capacity to alter the particular DNA succession liable for the illness could prepare for a fix or essentially ease its belongings. Clinical preliminaries and continuous examination are effectively investigating the remedial capability of CRISPR in tending to a range of hereditary problems.

In the domain of farming, CRISPR innovation has ignited another period of accuracy reproducing. The capacity to alter the genomes of yields holds enormous commitment for improving rural efficiency and maintainability. Researchers are chipping away at creating crops with further developed protection from irritations, illnesses, and ecological stressors. Furthermore, the change of yields for upgraded healthful substance is a center region, addressing worldwide difficulties connected with food security and lack of healthy sustenance.

Domesticated animals is likewise an objective for hereditary change utilizing CRISPR innovation. The capacity to present explicit hereditary changes can prompt creatures with upgraded qualities, like superior infection opposition or expanded meat and milk creation. Be that as it may, the use of quality altering in farming raises moral contemplations and worries about the possible long haul influences on biological systems and biodiversity.

In the field of malignant growth research, CRISPR innovation is assuming a critical part in propelling comprehension we might interpret the sickness and creating novel remedial procedures. Analysts can utilize CRISPR to target and alter qualities related with malignant growth, preparing for more exact and customized disease medicines. The innovation has likewise worked with the production of complex creature models for concentrating on malignant growth, empowering analysts to investigate the complexities of the infection and test expected mediations.

While the capability of CRISPR innovation in treating hereditary sicknesses and propelling horticulture is promising, it isn't without its moral contemplations. The possibility of controlling the human germline — changing the hereditary material that can be given to people in the future — brings up significant moral and moral issues. The capacity to alter the germline presents the chance of making heritable changes that could have sweeping outcomes, both planned and accidental.

The global academic local area has perceived the significance of tending to these moral worries and laying out clear rules for the capable utilization of CRISPR innovation. Gatherings and meetings have been assembled to cultivate conversations among researchers, ethicists, policymakers, and general society. Finding some kind of harmony between the possible advantages of quality altering and the moral contemplations encompassing its utilization is basic for the mindful progression of this progressive innovation.

The openness and effortlessness of CRISPR innovation have additionally led to worries about its likely abuse. The democratization of quality altering instruments has made them all the more generally accessible, raising the apparition of unapproved and possibly destructive use. The idea of "biohackers" endeavoring quality altering beyond customary exploration and clinical settings highlights the requirement for vigorous guidelines and oversight to moderate dangers and forestall potentially negative results.

The worldwide academic local area confronted a turning point in 2018 when Chinese researcher Dr. He Jiankui professed to have made the world's most memorable hereditarily altered children utilizing CRISPR innovation. This declaration set off boundless judgment and lighted a reestablished center around the requirement for moral rules and worldwide cooperation to direct the utilization of quality altering in people. The occurrence highlighted the significance of mindful exploration and the expected results of unregulated quality altering rehearses.

Specialized difficulties additionally go with the commitment of CRISPR innovation. Worries about askew impacts — occurrences where the Cas9 protein inadvertently alters DNA groupings other than the expected objective — have been a point of convergence of exploration. Researchers are effectively attempting to improve the accuracy of CRISPR innovation, limiting askew impacts to guarantee the security and precision of quality altering applications.

The advancement of option CRISPR frameworks, like CRISPR-Cas12 and CRISPR-Cas13, addresses one more boondocks in quality altering research. These frameworks offer special benefits, including different objective successions and the capacity to alter RNA instead of DNA. Investigating these elective frameworks gives specialists extra devices for explicit applications and addresses a portion of the restrictions related with the first CRISPR-Cas9 framework.

As the field of quality altering propels, the moral, legitimate, and social ramifications become progressively intricate. Worldwide coordinated effort and open exchange are fundamental for address these difficulties and foster a system that guarantees the mindful and moral utilization of quality altering instruments. The requirement for a complete way to deal with moral contemplations is highlighted by verifiable points of reference, for example, the Asilomar Gathering on Recombinant DNA in 1975, which laid out rules for the protected utilization of recombinant DNA innovation.

The potential for CRISPR innovation to be utilized in human upgrade and the making of "creator children" presents extra moral aspects. The possibility of choosing or changing explicit attributes in incipient organisms, for example, knowledge or actual appearance, raises worries about the cultural ramifications of such mediations. The moral talk stretches out past the specialized parts of quality altering to incorporate more extensive inquiries regarding the meaning of predictability and the possible effect on variety inside the human populace.

The idea of hereditary improvement prompts conversations about friendly imbalance, as people with admittance to quality altering advancements might possess the ability to upgrade their kids' credits. Moral contemplations encompassing the evenhanded conveyance of advantages and the potential for making a hereditarily separated society are integral to the capable investigation of hereditary improvement innovations.

The ramifications of quality altering stretch out past human applications and into the domain of protection science. CRISPR innovation offers possible answers for address difficulties connected with biodiversity misfortune and biological system well-being. Endeavors are in progress to investigate the utilization of quality altering to restore terminated species or upgrade the flexibility of jeopardized ones. The capacity to alter the genomes of organic entities for protection purposes holds guarantee for relieving the effects of environmental change and living space debasement.

Notwithstanding, the utilization of quality altering in protection additionally raises moral and natural worries. Bringing hereditarily adjusted creatures into regular biological systems could have unseen side-effects, disturbing natural adjusts and cooperations. The potential for biological mischief and the moral ramifications of changing the hereditary cosmetics of species in the wild require cautious thought and careful gamble appraisal prior to executing quality altering procedures in preservation rehearses.

In the lawful space, the quick advancement in quality altering has outperformed the improvement of complete administrative systems. The current administrative scene changes across nations, prompting an absence of normalized rules for the moral and capable utilization of CRISPR innovation. The shortfall of fit global guidelines brings difficulties up in guaranteeing a reliable and generally relevant structure that considers different moral, social, and cultural viewpoints.

Protection and security concerns likewise go with the ascent of quality altering advancements. The capacity to control the hereditary code brings up issues about the likely abuse of hereditary data, including unapproved admittance to people's hereditary information and the gamble of hereditary segregation. Shielding hereditary protection and laying out secure conventions for dealing with hereditary data are basic contemplations as quality altering innovations become more common.

In the domain of irresistible illnesses, CRISPR innovation has arisen as a promising device for creating novel antiviral methodologies. Specialists are investigating the utilization of CRISPR to target and cripple viral genomes, offering another way to deal with fighting viral contaminations. The flexibility of CRISPR innovation considers the fast improvement of designated antiviral treatments, giving an expected device in the continuous fight against arising viral dangers.

The intermingling of CRISPR innovation and computerized reasoning (simulated intelligence) holds the possibility to speed up examination and improve the effectiveness of quality altering processes. Artificial intelligence calculations can break down tremendous datasets, foresee potential off-target impacts, and improve CRISPR plans, smoothing out the exploratory work process. The collaboration among simulated intelligence and CRISPR innovation represents the interdisciplinary idea of present day logical exploration and its ability to drive development across assorted fields.

While moral conversations principally center around human and creature utilizations of quality altering, the utilization of CRISPR innovation in microorganisms presents its own arrangement of contemplations. The potential for quality altering to be applied in the adjustment of microbes and different microorganisms for modern or ecological purposes opens new outskirts. Designed microorganisms with enhanced metabolic pathways can add to additional manageable and effective modern cycles.

In the modern area, quality altering can upgrade the creation of biofuels, catalysts, and other important bioproducts. Designed microorganisms with enhanced metabolic pathways can add to additional manageable and effective modern cycles. In any case, the arrival of hereditarily altered microorganisms into the climate raises biological worries and requires cautious gamble evaluation to forestall potentially negative side-effects.

Ecological uses of quality altering reach out to the field of manufactured science, where microorganisms are intended for explicit capabilities, like natural remediation or the evacuation of poisons. The possible advantages of involving quality altered microorganisms for natural reclamation should be weighed against the likely dangers and potentially negative side-effects, stressing the significance of a prudent methodology in the use of quality altering techniques in ecological settings.

5.2 Potential applications for cancer treatment

The expected uses of quality altering and CRISPR innovation in malignant growth therapy have arisen as a promising boondocks in biomedical exploration. The many-sided nature of malignant growth, portrayed by hereditary transformations and modifications, makes it a great possibility for the accuracy and customization presented by CRISPR instruments. Specialists are investigating different systems to use CRISPR innovation in grasping the sub-atomic premise of disease, creating designated treatments, and progressing customized medication.

One of the essential utilizations of CRISPR in malignant growth research is the distinguishing proof and approval of disease related qualities. Extensive CRISPR screens empower analysts to methodicallly target and knockout qualities to notice their consequences for disease cell development and endurance. This approach uncovers the hereditary drivers of disease and recognize possible remedial targets. By understanding the particular qualities that add to the turn of events and movement of disease, specialists can foster more designated and successful medicines.

CRISPR innovation likewise assumes an essential part in making modern cell and creature models for concentrating on disease. Customary malignant growth models frequently miss the mark in precisely restating the intricacy of human cancers. With CRISPR, analysts can unequivocally bring disease related transformations into the genomes of cells or creatures, emulating the hereditary scene of human tumors all the more intently.

These hereditarily designed models give important bits of knowledge into malignant growth science, permitting analysts to test new treatments and review the basic systems of the illness.

In the domain of immunotherapy, CRISPR has opened new roads for upgrading the viability of resistant based malignant growth medicines. Fanciful Antigen Receptor (Vehicle) Lymphocyte treatment, a type of immunotherapy, includes changing a patient's own insusceptible cells to perceive and target disease cells. CRISPR innovation considers the exact designing of White blood cells to communicate Vehicles that explicitly target disease related antigens. This customization upgrades the restorative capability of Vehicle Lymphocyte treatment, making it more specific and powerful in going after disease cells while limiting damage to sound cells.

Past Vehicle White blood cell treatment, CRISPR is additionally being utilized to work on the viability of other immunotherapeutic methodologies, like safe designated spot inhibitors. By altering qualities engaged with invulnerable guideline, analysts plan to improve the insusceptible framework's capacity to perceive and kill malignant growth cells. The blend of CRISPR innovation with immunotherapy holds guarantee for growing more powerful and customized malignant growth medicines.

The capacity of CRISPR to target explicit qualities ensnared in disease movement has prepared for the advancement of novel remedial systems. Analysts are investigating quality altering to straightforwardly target and disturb the capability of oncogenes — qualities that drive disease development. By crippling these oncogenes, CRISPR innovation can possibly stop or dial back the uncontrolled multiplication of disease cells. This approach addresses a change in perspective in malignant growth treatment, moving towards mediations at the hereditary level to address the underlying drivers of the sickness.

Growth silencer qualities, which regularly capability to forestall the improvement of disease, can likewise be designated utilizing CRISPR innovation. By reestablishing the capability of inactivated cancer silencer qualities, analysts mean to restore the normal systems that control cell development and forestall the arrangement of growths. This approach holds guarantee for creating treatments that can return the hereditary changes driving malignant growth, possibly prompting more solid and manageable treatment results.

Chasing after accuracy medication, CRISPR innovation empowers the advancement of customized malignant growth treatments custom-made to the remarkable hereditary profile of every patient's cancer. Patient-determined xenografts (PDX) models, produced by relocating human malignant growth cells into creature has, can be altered utilizing CRISPR to recreate the particular hereditary changes present in a patient's growth. This permits scientists to test the responsiveness of individual cancers to various therapies, preparing for customized restorative procedures.

The adaptability of CRISPR innovation reaches out to the change of disease cells for restorative purposes. With regards to supportive cell treatments, where a patient's own insusceptible cells are designed to target and obliterate disease cells, CRISPR works with the exact altering of these phones. Analysts can improve the restorative capability of assenting cell treatments by changing safe cells to oppose fatigue, persevere longer in the body, and display expanded enemy of disease action.

CRISPR-interceded genome altering likewise holds guarantee for defeating difficulties related with conventional disease therapies, like chemotherapy and radiation treatment. By altering the qualities answerable for drug opposition, analysts intend to sharpen malignant growth cells to chemotherapy, making them more vulnerable with the impacts of against disease drugs. Moreover, CRISPR can be utilized to upgrade the accuracy of radiation treatment by specifically focusing on and adjusting qualities associated with the DNA fix instruments of disease cells.

The coming of CRISPR innovation has sped up the advancement of oncolytic infections — infections that specifically contaminate and annihilate malignant growth cells while saving ordinary cells. By altering the viral genome utilizing CRISPR, analysts can improve the growth focusing on capacities of oncolytic infections and limit their off-target impacts. This approach addresses a novel and possibly powerful technique for malignant growth therapy, utilizing the innate capacity of infections to imitate in and obliterate disease cells specifically.

Notwithstanding the huge capability of CRISPR innovation in malignant growth treatment, a few difficulties and contemplations should be tended to. One huge obstacle is the proficient conveyance of CRISPR parts to malignant growth cells inside the body. The improvement of compelling and safe conveyance techniques, like viral vectors or nanoparticles, is urgent for interpreting CRISPR-based disease treatments from the research facility to the center.

Off-target impacts, where CRISPR incidentally alters qualities other than the expected objective, stay a worry. Techniques to upgrade the explicitness of CRISPR, for example, the utilization of improved Cas9 variations and bioinformatics apparatuses for anticipating askew impacts, are effectively being sought after. Thorough testing and approval of CRISPR-altered cells and living beings are fundamental to guarantee the exactness and wellbeing of helpful mediations.

Moral contemplations additionally go with the utilization of CRISPR innovation in disease treatment. The potential for germline altering, where heritable changes are brought into the DNA of people in the future, brings up significant moral and cultural issues. Mindful and straightforward administration systems should be laid out to direct the moral utilization of CRISPR in malignant growth exploration and treatment, adjusting the quest for logical progressions with the need to safeguard people and maintain cultural qualities.

The developing scene of CRISPR-based malignant growth treatments features the powerful idea of biomedical examination and the continuous mission for inventive answers for complex clinical difficulties. As specialists keep on unwinding the hereditary complexities of malignant growth and foster progressively refined quality altering apparatuses, the possibility of extraordinary and customized disease medicines moves nearer to the real world. The joining of CRISPR innovation into the munititions stockpile of disease treatments holds the possibility to alter the field, offering new desire to patients and reshaping the worldview of malignant growth care.

5.3 Ethical considerations and challenges associated with gene editing

Quality altering advances, especially CRISPR (Bunched Consistently Interspaced Short Palindromic Rehashes), have introduced another time of logical conceivable outcomes, yet they likewise deliver a horde of moral contemplations and difficulties. As specialists bridle the ability to unequivocally change the hereditary code of living organic entities, a scope of moral difficulties arises, traversing from the expected abuse of the innovation to major inquiries concerning modifying the human germline.

One of the preeminent moral worries in the domain of quality altering spins around the idea of "fashioner children." This includes choosing or changing explicit characteristics in incipient organisms, going from actual traits to likely improvements in knowledge or other mental capacities. The possibility of making hereditarily designed people brings up moral issues about the commodification of human qualities, the potential for social disparity in light of hereditary benefits, and the effect on the variety of the human populace.

The capacity to alter the human germline, which contains the hereditary material that can be given to people in the future, presents significant moral situations. Presenting heritable changes through quality altering has suggestions for the people being treated as well as for their relatives too. This brings up issues about the drawn out results, accidental impacts, and the obligation of researchers and society to consider the prosperity of people in the future.

The global academic local area perceives the gravity of these moral worries, provoking conversations and discussions about the mindful utilization of quality altering innovations. In 2018, the World Wellbeing Association (WHO) laid out a worldwide warning council on human genome altering, stressing the requirement for global collaboration to explore the moral elements of quality altering. The board intends to give direction on the administration of human genome altering, guaranteeing that moral contemplations are integral to the development of this innovation.

Another huge moral concern spins around the potential for unseen side-effects and off-target impacts related with quality altering. While CRISPR innovation is intended to definitively target explicit DNA successions, there is dependably a gamble of unexpected changes happening somewhere else in the genome.

The results of such askew impacts could go from harmless changes to additional serious disturbances of fundamental qualities, possibly prompting unexpected medical problems.

To address these worries, scientists are constantly refining and upgrading the accuracy of CRISPR innovation. High level Cas9 variations, bioinformatics apparatuses for anticipating askew impacts, and thorough testing conventions are being created to limit the dangers related with accidental hereditary changes. Be that as it may, the intrinsic intricacy of organic frameworks and the unique idea of hereditary collaborations make it trying to wipe out all potential off-target impacts completely.

The democratization of quality altering instruments additionally raises moral contemplations with respect to openness and control. The rising effortlessness and reasonableness of CRISPR innovation make it more open to a more extensive scope of people, including DIY biohackers and resident researchers. This availability raises worries about the potential for unapproved and possibly destructive utilization of quality altering outside the conventional limits of examination and clinical settings.

The Do-It-Yourself biohacking local area, comprising of people without formal logical preparation exploring different avenues regarding hereditary changes, presents extraordinary difficulties. While numerous individuals from this local area are driven by interest and a longing to investigate logical ideas, the absence of oversight and adherence to moral principles raises worries about wellbeing, potentially negative results, and the requirement for mindful utilization of quality altering innovations.

In 2018, the activities of Chinese researcher Dr. He Jiankui, who professed to have made the world's most memorable hereditarily altered infants utilizing CRISPR innovation, lighted a worldwide moral emergency. The examination, pointed toward giving protection from HIV, was generally censured for its absence of straightforwardness, insufficient thought of moral rules, and the unanticipated dangers it presented to the altered undeveloped organisms. The occurrence highlighted the desperation of laying out clear moral rules and worldwide joint effort to manage the utilization of quality altering in people.

The idea of "hereditary separation" is one more moral concern related with quality altering. As people get to data about their hereditary cosmetics, there is a gamble that this data could be utilized to victimize them in different settings, like work, protection, or social communications. Shielding hereditary protection and laying out legitimate systems to forestall hereditary segregation are fundamental parts of the moral contemplations encompassing quality altering.

Moral contemplations in quality altering reach out past people to envelop the treatment of creatures and the adjustment of environments. The utilization of CRISPR innovation in horticulture, for instance, brings up issues about the government assistance of hereditarily

changed organic entities (GMOs), the likely natural effects of delivering altered organic entities into the climate, and the more extensive moral ramifications of designing qualities in creatures for human advantage.

In the domain of preservation science, where quality altering holds the possibility to resuscitate terminated species or improve the flexibility of imperiled ones, moral contemplations are especially perplexing. Bringing hereditarily changed life forms into normal environments could upset biological equilibriums and connections, bringing up issues about the moral obligation of researchers to gauge the possible advantages against the dangers and potentially negative results cautiously.

The moral contemplations encompassing quality altering are not exclusively the space of researchers and policymakers; they additionally reach out to public discernment and commitment. Public mindfulness, understanding, and acknowledgment of quality altering advancements assume a significant part in molding the moral scene. Guaranteeing that the general population is very much educated, participated in conversations about the ramifications of quality altering, and has a voice in dynamic cycles are essential to laying out moral structures that line up with cultural qualities.

Strict and social points of view further add to the moral intricacy of quality altering. Different conviction frameworks have changing perspectives on the control of the hereditary code, the holiness of life, and the moral limits of mediating in the normal request. Exploring these different points of view requires a nuanced and comprehensive way to deal with moral thoughts that thinks about an expansive scope of social, strict, and philosophical perspectives.

As quality altering advancements keep on progressing, moral contemplations stay at the front of conversations in mainstream researchers and then some. Finding some kind of harmony between logical advancement, capable use, and moral standards is a continuous test that requires coordinated effort among researchers, ethicists, policymakers, and people in general. The advancement of extensive and universally perceived moral rules is vital for guide the capable utilization of quality altering innovations and guarantee that the potential advantages are acknowledged without compromising moral principles.

Quality altering innovations, especially the progressive CRISPR-Cas9 framework, have achieved extraordinary capacities to control the hereditary code of living organic entities. While these innovations hold huge commitment for propelling science, medication, and horticulture, they likewise lead to a heap of moral contemplations. As scientists dig into the complexities of quality altering, investigating its expected applications and suggestions, moral difficulties arise across different areas, enveloping human wellbeing, horticulture, protection, and cultural standards.

With regards to human quality altering, one of the essential moral contemplations rotates around the idea of germline altering. Germline altering includes adjusting the DNA of incipient organisms or regenerative cells, presenting heritable changes that can be given to people in the future. While this approach holds the possibility to wipe out hereditary infections and issues from the germline, it brings up significant moral issues about the changelessness of hereditary modifications, the unexpected ramifications for people in the future, and the cultural obligation to go with choices that influence the human genetic stock.

The possibility of "fashioner infants," wherein explicit attributes like insight, actual appearance, or athletic ability can be chosen or improved through quality altering, presents moral intricacies. The possibility of controlling the hereditary cosmetics of people for non-helpful purposes prompts worries about making a general public with foreordained qualities, compounding social disparities, and testing the standards of hereditary variety and human independence.

The global academic local area recognizes the gravity of germline altering and has taken part in conversations to lay out moral rules. The Asilomar Meeting on Recombinant DNA in 1975 fills in as a verifiable point of reference, underlining the significance of capable exploration and the requirement for shields in hereditary designing. Worldwide cooperation is critical to foster universally perceived moral norms that guide the capable utilization of germline altering innovations, finding some kind of harmony between logical advancement and moral contemplations.

One more moral element of human quality altering concerns the idea of informed assent. As quality altering advances progress, the potential for hereditary mediations in people brings up issues about the straightforwardness of data gave to people taking part in clinical preliminaries or clinical medicines. Guaranteeing that people are enough educated about the dangers, advantages, and vulnerabilities related with quality altering intercessions is a key moral necessity, underscoring the significance of independence and regard for the decisions of those included.

Availability and value in the utilization of quality altering advances likewise present moral difficulties. As these advancements become more inescapable, concerns emerge about the potential for making incongruities between people or networks with admittance to state of the art hereditary intercessions and those without. Moral contemplations reach out to the worldwide circulation of advantages and dangers related with quality altering, accentuating the requirement for mindful and impartial admittance to arising hereditary treatments.

The idea of "biohackers" or DIY (Do-It-Yourself) hereditary designers presents novel moral difficulties. The rising openness and effortlessness of quality altering apparatuses empower people without formal logical preparation to participate in hereditary trial and error.

While the Do-It-Yourself biohacking local area is described by interest and a longing to investigate logical ideas, the absence of oversight raises worries about wellbeing, the potential for unseen side-effects, and the moral obligation of those directing hereditary tests outside customary exploration settings.

The 2018 instance of Chinese researcher Dr. He Jiankui, who professed to have made the world's most memorable hereditarily altered infants utilizing CRISPR, represents the moral difficulties related with the unregulated utilization of quality altering. Dr. He's analysis, pointed toward presenting protection from HIV, was broadly denounced for its absence of straightforwardness, deficient thought of moral rules, and the unanticipated dangers it presented to the altered undeveloped organisms. This episode highlighted the basic for severe guidelines and global coordinated effort to oversee the utilization of quality altering in people.

In agribusiness, the use of quality altering advancements brings up moral issues connected with hereditarily adjusted organic entities (GMOs) and the likely effects on environments. CRISPR innovation considers exact alterations to the genomes of harvests, offering the possibility of expanded versatility to illnesses, worked on nourishing substance, and improved rural efficiency. Nonetheless, worries about the accidental biological results of delivering hereditarily altered organic entities into the climate and the potential for hereditary defilement raise moral contemplations that warrant cautious assessment.

The moral components of horticultural quality altering additionally stretch out to issues of straightforwardness, public mindfulness, and the evenhanded dispersion of advantages. The's comprehension public might interpret quality altering in horticulture, including its possible advantages and dangers, is urgent for informed navigation. Moral contemplations request straightforwardness in the turn of events and organization of quality altered crops, with an emphasis on drawing in people in general in conversations about the moral ramifications of modifying the hereditary cosmetics of the food supply.

Preservation science faces moral difficulties with regards to utilizing quality altering to address biodiversity misfortune and biological system wellbeing. The possibility to resuscitate wiped out species or upgrade the strength of jeopardized ones through quality altering presents complex moral contemplations. The arrival of hereditarily adjusted creatures into regular biological systems could upset environmental equilibriums, presenting dangers to different species and living spaces. The moral obligation to painstakingly gauge the likely advantages against the dangers and unseen side-effects is fundamental in the utilization of quality altering in preservation.

The moral talk encompassing quality altering envelops the treatment of creatures, both with regards to farming and preservation. In agribusiness, quality altering offers the chance of improving the wellbeing, efficiency, and prosperity of animals.

In any case, worries about creature government assistance, the potential for unseen side-effects of hereditary alterations, and the drawn out influences on the biological systems where these creatures exist raise moral contemplations that require cautious assessment and moral oversight.

In the domain of preservation, the possibility to alter the genomes of creatures for protection purposes brings up moral issues about mediating in normal cycles. The utilization of quality altering to upgrade the flexibility of imperiled species or address dangers, for example, environmental change and territory misfortune requires a sensitive harmony between the moral basic to protect biodiversity and the potential natural dangers related with hereditary intercessions.

The lawful and administrative scene encompassing quality altering presents its own arrangement of moral difficulties. The fast progression of quality altering advances has outperformed the improvement of complete administrative structures. This absence of normalized rules and guidelines across various nations raises worries about the moral and capable utilization of quality altering. Worldwide coordinated effort is fundamental to lay out an orchestrated administrative structure that considers different moral, social, and cultural points of view encompassing quality altering.

Protection and security concerns additionally go with the ascent of quality altering innovations. The capacity to control the hereditary code brings up issues about the possible abuse of hereditary data, including unapproved admittance to people's hereditary information and the gamble of hereditary separation. Shielding hereditary protection and laying out secure conventions for taking care of hereditary data are basic contemplations as quality altering advancements become more common.

Moral contemplations reach out past the specialized parts of quality altering to more extensive inquiries concerning cultural qualities, social standards, and the ramifications of modifying the basic structure blocks of life. Public commitment and exchange are fundamental parts of moral dynamic in quality altering, guaranteeing that assorted points of view are thought of, and choices line up with cultural qualities.

As quality altering advances keep on progressing, moral contemplations stay at the very front of conversations in established researchers and then some. Finding some kind of harmony between logical development, mindful use, and moral standards is a continuous test that requires coordinated effort among researchers, ethicists, policymakers, and the general population. The advancement of far reaching and universally perceived moral rules is vital for guide the dependable utilization of quality altering innovations and guarantee that the potential advantages are acknowledged without compromising moral norms.

Chapter 6

Nanotechnology in Cancer Treatment

Nanotechnology has arisen as an earth shattering field with the possibility to change different enterprises, including medication. Lately, scientists have progressively investigated the utilization of nanotechnology in the field of malignant growth treatment, looking for additional successful and designated ways to deal with battle this perplexing and decimating illness. The remarkable properties of nanomaterials, like their size, surface region, and reactivity, make them ideal contender for conveying helpful specialists straightforwardly to disease cells while limiting harm to sound tissues.

One of the critical difficulties in conventional disease therapies, like chemotherapy and radiation treatment, lies in their absence of explicitness. These therapies frequently hurt solid cells alongside carcinogenic ones, prompting serious incidental effects and decreasing the patient's personal satisfaction. Nanotechnology offers a promising answer for this issue by empowering the plan and creation of nanoparticles that can specifically target disease cells.

Nanoparticles can be designed to have explicit properties that improve their collaboration with malignant growth cells. For instance, the improved penetrability and maintenance (EPR) impact permits nanoparticles to amass specially in the growth tissue because of its broken veins and hindered lymphatic seepage. This inactive focusing on system exploits the extraordinary microenvironment of growths, working on the conveyance of helpful specialists to disease cells while saving sound tissues.

Dynamic focusing on techniques further improve the accuracy of nanoparticle-based disease treatments. Ligands, like antibodies or peptides, can be connected to the outer layer of nanoparticles to perceive and tie to explicit receptors on disease cells. This dynamic focusing on approach expands the take-up of nanoparticles by malignant growth cells, advancing a more successful and limited treatment.

The adaptability of nanomaterials likewise takes into consideration the synchronous conveyance of numerous helpful specialists. This capacity is especially important in malignant growth treatment, where a blend of medications might be more powerful than single-specialist treatments. Nanoparticles can embody chemotherapeutic medications, nucleic acids, and imaging specialists, making multifunctional stages that empower both analysis and treatment.

In the domain of disease conclusion, nanotechnology plays had a crucial impact in propelling imaging procedures. Contrast specialists in view of nanomaterials upgrade the responsiveness and explicitness of imaging modalities, for example, attractive reverberation imaging (X-ray), processed tomography (CT), and positron outflow tomography (PET). These nanomaterial-based contrast specialists work on the representation of growths, helping with early recognition and precise organizing of disease.

Nanotechnology has additionally added to the improvement of imaginative malignant growth treatments, for example, photothermal treatment (PTT) and photodynamic treatment (PDT). In PTT, nanoparticles assimilate light and convert it into heat, specifically annihilating disease cells through hyperthermia. In the mean time, PDT includes the actuation of photosensitizing specialists by light, prompting the development of receptive oxygen species that prompt disease cell passing. The designated idea of these treatments limits harm to encompassing sound tissues, offering a more specific and less obtrusive treatment choice.

The utilization of nanotechnology in disease treatment stretches out past the domain of customary treatments. Nanoparticles can act as transporters for quality conveyance, opening up new roads for quality treatment in malignant growth. Quality treatment expects to address the basic hereditary anomalies that add to disease advancement and movement. By conveying helpful qualities to malignant growth cells, nanocarriers empower the tweak of quality articulation, advancing apoptosis, repressing angiogenesis, and upgrading the body's invulnerable reaction against disease.

The safe framework assumes a significant part in malignant growth observation and protection. In any case, disease cells can avoid safe discovery and annihilation through different systems. Nanotechnology offers procedures to tackle the safe framework's power in the battle against disease. Nanoparticles can be intended to invigorate the insusceptible reaction by conveying antigens, adjuvants, or safe designated spot inhibitors. These immunomodulatory nanoparticles actuate and upgrade the counter growth insusceptible reaction, possibly prompting more solid and fundamental impacts.

The improvement of nanovaccines addresses a promising way to deal with disease immunotherapy. Nanoparticles stacked with growth antigens and invulnerable invigorating particles mirror the attributes of microorganisms, actually preparing the resistant framework to perceive and go after disease cells. This customized and designated immunotherapeutic methodology holds extraordinary potential for treating different malignant growths, especially those with restricted reaction to ordinary treatments.

In spite of the colossal commitment of nanotechnology in malignant growth treatment, a few difficulties should be addressed to decipher these imaginative methodologies from the research facility to the center. One basic thought is the security of nanomaterials, as their cooperations with organic frameworks are mind boggling and diverse. Far reaching concentrates on the biocompatibility, pharmacokinetics, and long haul impacts of nanoparticles are fundamental to guarantee their protected use in malignant growth patients.

The expected harmfulness of nanomaterials raises worries about their effect on solid tissues and organs. Specialists are effectively investigating methodologies to alleviate poisonousness, like surface alteration and the utilization of biocompatible materials. Understanding the destiny of nanoparticles in the body, including their dissemination, digestion, and discharge, is significant for anticipating and limiting any antagonistic impacts.

The insusceptible framework's reaction to nanomaterials is another viewpoint that requires cautious thought. The body's safeguard instruments might perceive nanoparticles as unfamiliar intruders, prompting resistant actuation and likely freedom of the nanoparticles before they arrive at the growth site. Surface designing and alterations can assist with avoiding resistant acknowledgment, drawing out the flow season of nanoparticles and upgrading their collection in growths.

Moreover, the heterogeneity of cancers represents a test to nanotechnology-based therapies. Growths shift concerning size, morphology, and atomic qualities, making it trying to plan widespread nanoparticle stages that actually focus on a wide range of disease. Customized and versatile methodologies that consider the particular credits of individual growths are important to advance the adequacy of nanotechnology-based treatments.

Administrative contemplations likewise assume a significant part in the interpretation of nanotechnology from the research facility to clinical applications. The endorsement interaction for nanomedicines includes thorough appraisal of their security, adequacy, and assembling processes. Cooperation between scientists, administrative organizations, and industry partners is fundamental to lay out clear rules and principles for the turn of events and commercialization of nanotechnology-based disease medicines.

The monetary plausibility of nanotechnology-based disease treatments is one more element that impacts their reception in clinical practice. The expense of creating and delivering nanomedicines, as well as the framework expected for their organization, can influence their openness to patients. Monetary assessments and wellbeing innovation evaluations are fundamental parts of the dynamic interaction for medical services suppliers and policymakers thinking about the combination of nanotechnology into disease therapy conventions.

Regardless of these difficulties, the quick advancement in nanotechnology has prompted the improvement of various nanomedicines with promising preclinical and clinical outcomes. A few nanoparticle-based plans have entered clinical preliminaries, exhibiting their wellbeing and viability in different disease types. These preliminaries give significant bits of knowledge into this present reality pertinence of nanotechnology in disease treatment and add to the refinement of helpful systems.

In the domain of nanomedicine, liposomes address one of the earliest and best nanoparticle stages. Liposomal definitions exemplify remedial specialists, for example, chemotherapeutic medications, inside a lipid bilayer. This plan further develops drug dissolvability, solidness, and flow time while taking into consideration controlled discharge at the objective site. Doxil, a liposomal plan of doxorubicin, was one of the first nanomedicines supported by the U.S. Food and Medication Organization (FDA) for the therapy of bosom malignant growth, ovarian disease, and Kaposi's sarcoma.

Polymeric nanoparticles, one more broadly investigated stage, offer the benefit of adaptability in plan and functionalization. These nanoparticles can be designed to exemplify different medications and display controlled drug discharge profiles. Abraxane, a nanoparticle egg whites bound paclitaxel detailing, has been supported for the therapy of bosom malignant growth, exhibiting the capability of polymeric nanoparticles in working on the helpful record of chemotherapy.

Inorganic nanoparticles, for example, gold and iron oxide nanoparticles, have one of a kind physical and substance properties that make them alluring for disease treatment. Gold nanoparticles, for example, show solid surface plasmon reverberation, permitting them to assimilate and change over light into heat for photothermal treatment. Iron oxide nanoparticles, then again, can act as difference specialists for imaging and as transporters for drug conveyance.

The field of nanomedicine has additionally seen the development of nucleic corrosive based therapeutics, including little meddling RNA (siRNA) and courier RNA (mRNA). These nucleic acids can be utilized to quietness explicit qualities or incite the statement of helpful proteins inside disease cells. Nanoparticle transporters shield nucleic acids from debasement and work with their conveyance to the objective site. The FDA endorsement of Onpattro, a lipid nanoparticle plan conveying siRNA for the treatment of inherited transthyretin-interceded amyloidosis, features the capability of nucleic corrosive based nanomedicines.

The combination of nanotechnology and immunotherapy has led to creative methodologies for upgrading the insusceptible framework's capacity to perceive and take out disease cells. Insusceptible designated spot inhibitors, like enemy of PD-1 and hostile to CTLA-4 antibodies, have upset disease treatment by releasing the resistant framework's enemy of cancer reactions. Nanoparticle-based conveyance frameworks can work on the pharmacokinetics and biodistribution of these immunotherapeutics, upgrading their helpful viability.

Dendrimers, exceptionally extended macromolecules with clear cut structures, address one more class of nanomaterials investigated for disease treatment. Dendrimers can be designed to convey drugs, imaging specialists, and focusing on ligands in a controlled and measured style. Their remarkable properties, including multivalency and high surface usefulness, make them reasonable for different applications in disease determination and treatment.

Carbon-based nanomaterials, like carbon nanotubes and graphene, stand out for their remarkable physicochemical properties. These materials can be functionalized and utilized for drug conveyance, imaging, and photothermal treatment. Notwithstanding, worries about their biocompatibility and long haul wellbeing should be entirely tended to before their boundless clinical application.

The joining of nanotechnology with accuracy medication approaches holds incredible commitment for fitting disease medicines to individual patients. Accuracy medication plans to recognize explicit sub-atomic changes in a patient's growth and coordinate them with designated treatments. Nanoparticles can be intended to convey designated treatments, including little particle inhibitors and monoclonal antibodies, straightforwardly to malignant growth cells holding onto explicit sub-atomic markers.

The capability of nanotechnology in accuracy medication is exemplified by the improvement of friend diagnostics, which empower the recognizable proof of patients who are probably going to profit from a specific treatment. These diagnostics, frequently founded on imaging or atomic profiling, guide the determination of proper nanomedicines or designated treatments, expanding treatment adequacy while limiting incidental effects.

The utilization of nanotechnology in malignant growth treatment stretches out to the domain of theranostics, a field that consolidates remedial and demonstrative capacities in a solitary stage. Nanotheranostics expect to incorporate imaging specialists with restorative specialists, taking into consideration continuous checking of treatment reaction. This approach works with customized treatment regimens, as clinicians can change treatment in view of the noticed restorative impacts.

Multifunctional nanoparticles furnished with imaging abilities add to the expanding field of picture directed treatment. These nanoparticles empower painless imaging of growths, directing the exact conveyance of remedial specialists to the objective site. Continuous observing of therapy reaction and early discovery of potential inconveniences improve the general adequacy of disease treatment.

The approach of nanotechnology in malignant growth therapy has likewise prodded headways in the field of oncotheranostics, which centers around joining disease treatment with synchronous checking of treatment reaction. Oncotheranostic approaches influence the interesting properties of nanomaterials to foster imaging specialists that give experiences into the atomic and practical changes happening inside cancers during therapy.

The improvement of customized nanomedicines requires a profound comprehension of the sub-atomic qualities of individual growths. Propels in omics advances, like genomics, proteomics, and metabolomics, have worked with the distinguishing proof of explicit biomarkers related with disease subtypes and treatment reaction. Incorporating these atomic bits of knowledge with nanotechnology considers the plan of custom fitted remedial procedures that address the remarkable highlights of every patient's malignant growth.

The potential for joining nanotechnology with other arising advancements, like man-made reasoning (computer based intelligence), holds incredible commitment for propelling disease treatment. Man-made intelligence calculations can dissect tremendous datasets, including genomic profiles, imaging information, and clinical records, to recognize examples and connections that might direct treatment choices. Nanotechnology, with its capacity to convey designated treatments and imaging specialists, adjusts synergistically with computer based intelligence driven accuracy medication draws near.

6.1 Overview of nanotechnology and its role in cancer treatment

Nanotechnology, a multidisciplinary field at the crossing point of material science, science, science, and designing, has collected critical consideration for changing different enterprises, including medicine potential. At the center of nanotechnology is the control and control of materials at the nanoscale, normally characterized as aspects going from 1 to 100 nanometers. This scale takes into consideration the double-dealing of exceptional physical and substance properties that emerge at such little aspects.

With regards to disease treatment, nanotechnology offers a promising and creative way to deal with address the impediments of customary treatments. Malignant growth, a mind boggling and heterogeneous infection, presents critical difficulties because of its capacity to dodge treatment and oppose helpful mediations. The ordinary techniques for chemotherapy and radiation treatment, while viable somewhat, frequently need particularity and can hurt sound tissues alongside disease cells, prompting serious secondary effects.

The utilization of nanotechnology in malignant growth therapy expects to conquer these difficulties by giving a stage to the plan and creation of nanomaterials that can specifically target disease cells while limiting harm to encompassing solid tissues. The remarkable properties of nanomaterials, like their little size, high surface region, and tunable surface science, make them ideal contender for conveying remedial specialists with accuracy and proficiency.

One of the basic standards fundamental the utilization of nanotechnology in disease treatment is the idea of designated drug conveyance. Conventional chemotherapy drugs flow all through the body, influencing both destructive and sound cells, prompting fundamental harmfulness. Nanoparticles, then again, can be designed to convey remedial specialists in a controlled way, considering designated conveyance to the growth site.

The improved porousness and maintenance (EPR) impact is a urgent peculiarity taken advantage of in nanotechnology-based drug conveyance for malignant growth treatment. Growths frequently display broken veins and impeded lymphatic waste, prompting the amassing of nanoparticles in the cancer microenvironment. This latent focusing on component exploits the unmistakable qualities of growths, permitting nanoparticles to amass in destructive tissues specially.

Notwithstanding inactive focusing on, dynamic focusing on systems further upgrade the accuracy of nanotechnology-based malignant growth treatments. Ligands like antibodies, peptides, or aptamers can be appended to the outer layer of nanoparticles to perceive and tie to explicit receptors on malignant growth cells. This dynamic focusing on approach builds the take-up of nanoparticles by malignant growth cells, working on the general adequacy of the treatment.

The adaptability of nanomaterials empowers the concurrent conveyance of numerous restorative specialists. This capacity is especially significant in disease treatment, where a blend of medications might be more compelling than single-specialist treatments. Nanoparticles can embody chemotherapeutic medications, nucleic acids, and imaging specialists, making multifunctional stages that convey remedial payloads as well as consider painless observing of the treatment reaction.

In the domain of disease finding, nanotechnology plays had a crucial impact in propelling imaging strategies. Contrast specialists in light of nanomaterials upgrade the awareness and particularity of imaging modalities, for example, attractive reverberation imaging (X-ray), figured tomography (CT), and positron emanation tomography (PET). These nanomaterial-based contrast specialists work on the representation of growths, supporting early recognition and exact organizing of disease.

Nanotechnology has additionally added to the improvement of inventive disease treatments, for example, photothermal treatment (PTT) and photodynamic treatment (PDT). In PTT, nanoparticles assimilate light and convert it into heat, specifically annihilating disease cells through hyperthermia. In the mean time, PDT includes the actuation of photosensitizing specialists by light, prompting the development of receptive oxygen species that actuate disease cell passing. The designated idea of these treatments limits harm to encompassing solid tissues, offering a more particular and less intrusive treatment choice.

The use of nanotechnology in malignant growth treatment reaches out past the domain of customary treatments. Nanoparticles can act as transporters for quality conveyance, opening up new roads for quality treatment in disease. Quality treatment plans to address the hidden hereditary irregularities that add to disease improvement and movement. By conveying remedial qualities to malignant growth cells, nanocarriers empower the balance of quality articulation, advancing apoptosis, hindering angiogenesis, and improving the body's invulnerable reaction against disease.

The safe framework assumes a urgent part in disease observation and protection. In any case, disease cells can sidestep resistant location and obliteration through different systems. Nanotechnology offers procedures to tackle the resistant framework's power in the battle against disease. Nanoparticles can be intended to invigorate the resistant reaction by conveying antigens, adjuvants, or invulnerable designated spot inhibitors.

These immunomodulatory nanoparticles enact and upgrade the counter cancer invulnerable reaction, possibly prompting more solid and fundamental impacts.

The improvement of nanovaccines addresses a promising way to deal with disease immunotherapy. Nanoparticles stacked with growth antigens and resistant animating atoms imitate the qualities of microbes, really preparing the invulnerable framework to perceive and go after disease cells. This customized and designated immunotherapeutic methodology holds extraordinary potential for treating various diseases, especially those with restricted reaction to traditional treatments.

Notwithstanding the gigantic commitment of nanotechnology in malignant growth treatment, a few difficulties should be addressed to decipher these imaginative methodologies from the research center to the facility.

One basic thought is the wellbeing of nanomaterials, as their connections with organic frameworks are mind boggling and complex. Extensive examinations on the biocompatibility, pharmacokinetics, and long haul impacts of nanoparticles are fundamental to guarantee their protected use in malignant growth patients.

The possible poisonousness of nanomaterials raises worries about their effect on sound tissues and organs. Scientists are effectively investigating techniques to relieve harmfulness, like surface change and the utilization of biocompatible materials. Understanding the destiny of nanoparticles in the body, including their dissemination, digestion, and discharge, is vital for anticipating and limiting any unfriendly impacts.

The invulnerable framework's reaction to nanomaterials is another perspective that requires cautious thought. The body's protection instruments might perceive nanoparticles as unfamiliar trespassers, prompting insusceptible enactment and possible leeway of the nanoparticles before they arrive at the growth site. Surface designing and adjustments can assist with dodging safe acknowledgment, dragging out the course season of nanoparticles and improving their amassing in growths.

Furthermore, the heterogeneity of cancers represents a test to nanotechnology-based therapies. Growths differ concerning size, morphology, and atomic qualities, making it trying to plan widespread nanoparticle stages that successfully focus on a wide range of disease. Customized and versatile methodologies that consider the particular ascribes of individual cancers are important to upgrade the adequacy of nanotechnology-based treatments.

Administrative contemplations likewise assume a pivotal part in the interpretation of nanotechnology from the lab to clinical applications. The endorsement cycle for nanomedicines includes thorough evaluation of their security, viability, and assembling processes. Coordinated effort between analysts, administrative organizations, and industry partners is fundamental to lay out clear rules and norms for the turn of events and commercialization of nanotechnology-based malignant growth medicines.

The monetary plausibility of nanotechnology-based disease treatments is one more variable that impacts their reception in clinical practice. The expense of creating and delivering nanomedicines, as well as the framework expected for their organization, can influence their openness to patients. Financial assessments and wellbeing innovation evaluations are imperative parts of the dynamic cycle for medical services suppliers and policymakers thinking about the joining of nanotechnology into malignant growth therapy conventions.

Notwithstanding these difficulties, the fast advancement in nanotechnology has prompted the improvement of various nanomedicines with promising preclinical and clinical outcomes. A few nanoparticle-based details have entered clinical preliminaries, exhibiting their security and viability in different malignant growth types.

These preliminaries give significant experiences into this present reality materialness of nanotechnology in disease treatment and add to the refinement of restorative techniques.

In the domain of nanomedicine, liposomes address one of the earliest and best nanoparticle stages. Liposomal details typify helpful specialists, for example, chemotherapeutic medications, inside a lipid bilayer. This plan further develops drug dissolvability, dependability, and dissemination time while taking into consideration controlled discharge at the objective site. Doxil, a liposomal definition of doxorubicin, was one of the first nanomedicines endorsed by the U.S. Food and Medication Organization (FDA) for the therapy of bosom disease, ovarian malignant growth, and Kaposi's sarcoma.

Polymeric nanoparticles, one more broadly investigated stage, offer the upside of adaptability in plan and functionalization. These nanoparticles can be designed to exemplify different medications and display controlled drug discharge profiles. Abraxane, a nanoparticle egg whites bound paclitaxel detailing, has been endorsed for the therapy of bosom malignant growth, exhibiting the capability of polymeric nanoparticles in working on the helpful record of chemotherapy.

Inorganic nanoparticles, for example, gold and iron oxide nanoparticles, have remarkable physical and substance properties that make them appealing for disease treatment. Gold nanoparticles, for example, show solid surface plasmon reverberation, permitting them to assimilate and change over light into heat for photothermal treatment. Iron oxide nanoparticles, then again, can act as difference specialists for imaging and as transporters for drug conveyance.

The field of nanomedicine has likewise seen the rise of nucleic corrosive based therapeutics, including little meddling RNA (siRNA) and courier RNA (mRNA). These nucleic acids can be utilized to quietness explicit qualities or initiate the declaration of restorative proteins inside malignant growth cells. Nanoparticle transporters shield nucleic acids from corruption and work with their conveyance to the objective site. The FDA endorsement of Onpattro, a lipid nanoparticle plan conveying siRNA for the treatment of innate transthyretin-interceded amyloidosis, features the capability of nucleic corrosive based nanomedicines.

The assembly of nanotechnology and immunotherapy has brought about imaginative methodologies for improving the resistant framework's capacity to perceive and kill disease cells. Resistant designated spot inhibitors, like enemy of PD-1 and against CTLA-4 antibodies, have changed malignant growth treatment by releasing the insusceptible framework's enemy of cancer reactions. Nanoparticle-based conveyance frameworks can work on the pharmacokinetics and biodistribution of these immunotherapeutics, upgrading their restorative adequacy.

Dendrimers, exceptionally stretched macromolecules with obvious designs, address one more class of nanomaterials investigated for disease treatment. Dendrimers can be designed to convey drugs, imaging specialists, and focusing on ligands in a controlled and particular style. Their special properties, including multivalency and high surface usefulness, make them reasonable for different applications in malignant growth analysis and treatment.

Carbon-based nanomaterials, like carbon nanotubes and graphene, stand out for their uncommon physicochemical properties. These materials can be functionalized and utilized for drug conveyance, imaging, and photothermal treatment. Nonetheless, worries about their biocompatibility and long haul security should be completely tended to before their inescapable clinical application.

The combination of nanotechnology with accuracy medication approaches holds extraordinary commitment for fitting malignant growth medicines to individual patients. Accuracy medication means to distinguish explicit sub-atomic modifications in a patient's cancer and coordinate them with designated treatments. Nanoparticles can be intended to convey designated treatments, including little atom inhibitors and monoclonal antibodies, straightforwardly to malignant growth cells holding onto explicit sub-atomic markers.

The capability of nanotechnology in accuracy medication is exemplified by the improvement of buddy diagnostics, which empower the ID of patients who are probably going to profit from a specific treatment. These diagnostics, frequently founded on imaging or sub-atomic profiling, guide the choice of proper nanomedicines or designated treatments, boosting treatment adequacy while limiting secondary effects.

The utilization of nanotechnology in disease treatment reaches out to the domain of theranostics, a field that joins restorative and symptomatic capacities in a solitary stage. Nanotheranostics intend to coordinate imaging specialists with helpful specialists, considering continuous observing of treatment reaction. This approach works with customized treatment regimens, as clinicians can change treatment in light of the noticed remedial impacts.

Multifunctional nanoparticles furnished with imaging capacities add to the thriving field of picture directed treatment. These nanoparticles empower harmless imaging of growths, directing the exact conveyance of helpful specialists to the objective site. Continuous observing of therapy reaction and early location of potential inconveniences improve the general adequacy of disease treatment.

The approach of nanotechnology in disease therapy has additionally prodded headways in the field of oncotheranostics, which centers around consolidating malignant growth treatment with concurrent checking of treatment reaction. Oncotheranostic approaches influence the special properties of nanomaterials to foster imaging specialists that give bits of knowledge into the sub-atomic and useful changes happening inside growths during treatment.

The improvement of customized nanomedicines requires a profound comprehension of the sub-atomic qualities of individual growths. Progresses in omics advances, like genomics, proteomics, and metabolomics, have worked with the recognizable proof of explicit biomarkers related with malignant growth subtypes and treatment reaction. Coordinating these atomic experiences with nanotechnology takes into consideration the plan of custom fitted helpful procedures that address the interesting elements of every patient's malignant growth.

The potential for joining nanotechnology with other arising innovations, like manmade brainpower (artificial intelligence), holds extraordinary commitment for propelling disease treatment. Artificial intelligence calculations can dissect tremendous datasets, including genomic profiles, imaging information, and clinical records, to distinguish examples and connections that might direct treatment choices. Nanotechnology, with its capacity to convey designated treatments and imaging specialists, adjusts synergistically with simulated intelligence driven accuracy medication draws near.

6.2 Nanoparticles and drug delivery systems

Nanoparticles and drug conveyance frameworks have reformed the scene of present day medication, offering imaginative answers for difficulties in drug conveyance, especially in the therapy of complicated sicknesses like disease. Nanoparticles, ordinarily going in size from 1 to 100 nanometers, have novel properties that make them profoundly appealing for designated drug conveyance. The capacity to design and tweak nanoparticles takes into account the exact conveyance of remedial specialists to explicit cells or tissues, amplifying helpful adequacy while limiting unfriendly impacts.

The field of medication conveyance has been changed by the coming of nanoparticles, which act as transporters for a different scope of restorative payloads, including little particles, proteins, nucleic acids, and imaging specialists. The plan of nanoparticles is directed by their expected application, with contemplations for size, surface science, and functionalization to upgrade their presentation in vivo.

One of the vital benefits of nanoparticles in drug conveyance lies in their capacity to latently target unhealthy tissues through the improved porousness and maintenance (EPR) impact. In malignant growth, for instance, cancers frequently display flawed vasculature, permitting nanoparticles to gather inside the growth microenvironment specifically. This inactive focusing on system has been utilized to work on the conveyance of chemotherapeutic specialists to disease cells while limiting openness to sound tissues.

Dynamic focusing on techniques further improve the accuracy of medication conveyance utilizing nanoparticles.

Ligands like antibodies, peptides, or aptamers can be formed to the outer layer of nanoparticles, granting explicitness for receptors overexpressed on the outer layer of target cells. This dynamic focusing on approach expands the take-up of nanoparticles by the ideal cells, working on the general restorative record of the conveyed drug.

Liposomes, a kind of nanoparticle, address one of the earliest and best medication conveyance frameworks. Liposomes are made out of lipid bilayers that embody hydrophilic or lipophilic medications, giving a flexible stage to tranquilize conveyance. Doxil, a liposomal plan of doxorubicin, represents the progress of liposomes in clinical applications, showing further developed wellbeing and viability contrasted with customary doxorubicin.

Polymeric nanoparticles, one more broadly investigated stage, offer benefits with regards to biocompatibility, dependability, and controlled drug discharge. These nanoparticles can be combined from regular or manufactured polymers, considering the epitome of different medications and their delivery in a controlled way. Abraxane, a nanoparticle egg whites bound paclitaxel plan, has been endorsed for the therapy of bosom disease, displaying the capability of polymeric nanoparticles in further developing medication dissolvability and conveyance.

Inorganic nanoparticles, including gold and iron oxide nanoparticles, have special physicochemical properties that make them appealing for drug conveyance and imaging. Gold nanoparticles, for example, display solid surface plasmon reverberation, permitting them to ingest and change over light into heat for photothermal treatment. Iron oxide nanoparticles can act as differentiation specialists for imaging and as transporters for drug conveyance. The multifunctionality of these inorganic nanoparticles makes them significant apparatuses in the advancement of theranostic stages.

Nanoparticles have likewise been utilized in the conveyance of nucleic corrosive based therapeutics, like little meddling RNA (siRNA) and courier RNA (mRNA). Nucleic corrosive based drugs have shown extraordinary commitment in regulating quality articulation for restorative purposes. In any case, their conveyance presents critical difficulties because of defenselessness to debasement and wasteful cell take-up. Nanoparticles safeguard nucleic acids and work with their conveyance to target cells, as exhibited by the FDA-supported lipid nanoparticle definition, Onpattro, for the treatment of innate transthyretin-intervened amyloidosis.

Carbon-based nanomaterials, like carbon nanotubes and graphene, have arisen as flexible stages for drug conveyance and imaging. These materials offer one of a kind physical and substance properties, including high surface region and electrical conductivity. Functionalized carbon nanotubes have been investigated for the conveyance of chemotherapeutic medications, while graphene oxide nanoparticles have shown guarantee in quality conveyance and photothermal treatment.

Dendrimers, profoundly fanned macromolecules with obvious designs, address one more class of nanomaterials with applications in drug conveyance. Dendrimers can be definitively designed to convey drugs, imaging specialists, and focusing on ligands in a controlled style. Their multivalent design considers the formation of numerous utilitarian gatherings, making them reasonable for different applications in drug conveyance and diagnostics.

The utilization of nanoparticles in drug conveyance isn't restricted to malignant growth treatment; it reaches out to many remedial regions, including irresistible illnesses, cardiovascular problems, and neurological circumstances. The capacity to tailor the properties of nanoparticles for explicit applications has prompted the improvement of designated treatments that address the interesting difficulties presented by various infections.

Notwithstanding the striking advancement in the field of nanoparticle-based drug conveyance, a few difficulties remain. One basic thought is the possible harmfulness of nanomaterials. The collaborations among nanoparticles and natural frameworks are perplexing, and far reaching concentrates on biocompatibility, pharmacokinetics, and long haul impacts are fundamental to guarantee the protected utilization of nanoparticles in clinical settings.

The resistant framework's reaction to nanoparticles is one more component that impacts their viability in drug conveyance. The body's protection components might perceive nanoparticles as unfamiliar intruders, prompting insusceptible enactment and possible leeway of the nanoparticles prior to arriving at the objective site. Surface adjustments and designing procedures are utilized to sidestep resistant acknowledgment, dragging out the course season of nanoparticles and improving their collection in ailing tissues.

The heterogeneity of sicknesses, especially on account of disease, represents a test to the improvement of general nanoparticle stages. Cancers differ regarding size, morphology, and atomic attributes, requiring customized and versatile ways to deal with enhance the viability of nanoparticle-based treatments. Accuracy medication, combined with progressions in diagnostics, considers the customization of nanoparticle definitions in light of individual patient profiles.

Administrative contemplations likewise assume a pivotal part in the interpretation of nanoparticle-based drug conveyance frameworks from the research center to clinical applications. The endorsement cycle for nanomedicines includes thorough appraisal of security, viability, and assembling processes. Coordinated effort between scientists, administrative organizations, and industry partners is fundamental to lay out clear rules and norms for the turn of events and commercialization of nanoparticle-based drug conveyance frameworks.

The monetary practicality of nanoparticle-based drug conveyance frameworks is one more element that impacts their reception in clinical practice. The expense of creating and delivering nanomedicines, as well as the framework expected for their organization, can influence their availability to patients.

Financial assessments and wellbeing innovation evaluations are essential parts of the dynamic interaction for medical services suppliers and policymakers considering the mix of nanoparticle-based drug conveyance frameworks into existing therapy conventions.

6.3 Current research and developments in nanomedicine

Flow exploration and improvements in nanomedicine are at the front of logical development, promising pivotal headways in the conclusion, treatment, and checking of different sicknesses. Nanomedicine, a multidisciplinary field that joins nanotechnology with medication, use the remarkable properties of nanomaterials to address difficulties in conventional restorative and symptomatic methodologies. From designated drug conveyance to imaging and then some, nanomedicine is ready to reshape the scene of medical care.

One area of dynamic exploration in nanomedicine is the improvement of designated drug conveyance frameworks that mean to upgrade the remedial adequacy of medications while limiting secondary effects. Nanoparticles, like liposomes, polymeric nanoparticles, and dendrimers, are designed to exemplify medicates and convey them specifically to unhealthy tissues. This designated drug conveyance approach holds specific commitment in disease therapy, where the test lies in specifically focusing on malignant growth cells while saving solid tissues.

As of late, specialists have investigated the utilization of nanoparticles for conveying various restorative specialists, including chemotherapeutic medications, nucleic acids, and immunomodulatory specialists. The multifunctionality of nanoparticles takes into account the co-conveyance of different medications, empowering blend treatments that might be more powerful than single-specialist medicines. For instance, nanocarriers can epitomize chemotherapeutic medications to target disease cells while at the same time conveying immunomodulatory specialists to upgrade the body's insusceptible reaction against the growth.

In the domain of malignant growth treatment, nanomedicine has additionally added to the advancement of imaginative medicines, for example, photothermal treatment (PTT) and photodynamic treatment (PDT). Nanoparticles, especially those containing materials like gold or photosensitizing specialists, can retain light and convert it into heat or receptive oxygen species, specifically obliterating disease cells. These light-set off treatments offer the benefit of confined treatment, limiting harm to encompassing solid tissues.

Nanomedicine is taking huge steps in the field of quality treatment, planning to address hereditary irregularities at the sub-atomic level. Nanoparticles act as transporters for nucleic corrosive based therapeutics, like little meddling RNA (siRNA) and courier RNA (mRNA), which can balance quality articulation. This approach holds guarantee for treating hereditary problems, as well concerning customized disease treatments focusing on unambiguous hereditary transformations inside cancers.

Imaging strategies assume a significant part in sickness finding and checking, and nanomedicine has added to the improvement of cutting edge imaging contrast specialists. Nanoparticles intended for imaging applications improve the responsiveness and explicitness of imaging modalities, for example, attractive reverberation imaging (X-ray), figured tomography (CT), and positron discharge tomography (PET). These difference specialists give better perception of ailing tissues, empowering early recognition and precise portrayal of sicknesses.

Moreover, theranostic nanoparticles, which incorporate both restorative and symptomatic functionalities, address a prospering area of examination. These multifunctional nanoparticles convey helpful specialists as well as empower ongoing observing of treatment reaction. Theranostic approaches can possibly tailor treatment regimens in view of individual patient reactions, preparing for customized medication.

The union of nanomedicine and immunotherapy has opened new roads for tackling the resistant framework's power in the battle against malignant growth and different illnesses. Nanoparticles can be designed to invigorate invulnerable reactions by conveying antigens, adjuvants, or safe designated spot inhibitors. This immunomodulatory job of nanoparticles improves the body's capacity to perceive and dispose of malignant growth cells, offering a foundational and solid way to deal with disease treatment.

Nanovaccines, a subset of immunotherapies, influence nanoparticles to emulate microbes and train the insusceptible framework to perceive and go after unambiguous antigens related with malignant growth or irresistible illnesses. These customized immunizations hold guarantee for prompting hearty and designated resistant reactions, possibly prompting further developed results in malignant growth patients and upgraded assurance against irresistible microbes.

In nervous system science, nanomedicine is taking huge steps in crossing the bloodmind obstruction, an impressive test in conveying therapeutics to the cerebrum. Nanoparticles intended to explore this obstruction might possibly convey medications to treat neurodegenerative infections, mind growths, and other neurological problems. The capacity to exactly target explicit locales inside the mind while limiting fundamental openness is a basic headway in the field of neurotherapeutics.

The incorporation of nanotechnology and regenerative medication has prompted the improvement of nanomaterials that help tissue recovery and fix. Nanoparticles can be designed to impersonate the extracellular grid and give a favorable climate to cell development and tissue recovery. This approach holds guarantee for treating conditions like degenerative joint sicknesses, spinal rope wounds, and cardiovascular problems.

In irresistible sickness the board, nanomedicine is adding to the advancement of imaginative antimicrobial specialists and immunizations. Nanoparticles can be functionalized with antimicrobial peptides or stacked with antimicrobial medications to battle drug-safe diseases. Moreover, nanovaccines offer a stage for designated conveyance of antigens to get strong insusceptible reactions against irresistible specialists, possibly upsetting immunization improvement.

While the capability of nanomedicine is immense, moves endure on the way to clinical interpretation. The wellbeing profile of nanomaterials, their drawn out impacts, and potential immunogenicity are basic contemplations that require intensive examination. Specialists are effectively attempting to address these worries through exhaustive preclinical examinations to guarantee the protected and viable utilization of nanomedicines in clinical settings.

Administrative endorsement cycles and normalization of assembling rehearses are pivotal for the fruitful interpretation of nanomedicine from the research center to clinical applications. Cooperative endeavors including analysts, administrative organizations, and industry accomplices are fundamental to lay out rules that guarantee the quality, security, and viability of nanomedicines.

Additionally, headways in nanomedicine are firmly entwined with the advancing scene of man-made reasoning (artificial intelligence) and AI. The incorporation of computer based intelligence calculations with nanomedicine information can work with the distinguishing proof of novel helpful targets, anticipate patient reactions, and enhance treatment regimens. This cooperative energy among nanotechnology and simulated intelligence holds the possibility to speed up drug disclosure and improve the accuracy of customized medication.

Chapter 7

Artificial Intelligence in Oncology

Computerized reasoning (man-made intelligence) has arisen as an extraordinary power across different enterprises, and medical services is no exemption. Specifically, simulated intelligence's applications in oncology have shown gigantic commitment in further developing determination, treatment arranging, and patient results. The reconciliation of man-made intelligence innovations into oncology rehearses can possibly upset how disease is perceived, analyzed, and treated.

One of the essential difficulties in oncology is the intricacy of disease itself. Malignant growth is a heterogeneous infection with different sub-atomic and hereditary profiles, presenting every defense special. Customary techniques for disease determination and treatment frequently depend on a one-size-fits-all methodology, which may not be ideal for each understanding. This is where computer based intelligence moves toward, offering the capacity to examine tremendous measures of information rapidly and proficiently, giving customized bits of knowledge and treatment choices.

The above all else utilization of man-made intelligence in oncology is in the domain of diagnostics. Computer based intelligence calculations can investigate clinical pictures, for example, X-beams, CT sweeps, and X-rays, with a degree of exactness and speed that outperforms human capacities. This can essentially diminish the time it takes to recognize growths and decide their qualities. For example, artificial intelligence fueled picture examination can recognize unpretentious examples or irregularities in clinical pictures that might be demonstrative of carcinogenic developments, empowering prior and more precise conclusion.

Besides, man-made intelligence assumes a critical part in genomics and sub-atomic examination, assisting scientists and clinicians with understanding the hidden hereditary transformations and modifications related with various kinds of malignant growths. This information is fundamental for fitting treatment methodologies to individual patients, introducing a time of accuracy medication. By utilizing simulated intelligence to decipher complex genomic information, oncologists can recognize explicit biomarkers that impact malignant growth improvement and reaction to treatment.

In the domain of treatment arranging, simulated intelligence helps oncologists in concocting customized and designated treatment plans. The coordination of patient information, including hereditary data, treatment history, and reaction to past treatments, permits artificial intelligence calculations to suggest the best treatment choices. This improves the possibilities of fruitful results as well as limits the gamble of unfriendly impacts by keeping away from medicines that are probably not going to be gainful.

The idea of virtual growth sheets is another region where man-made intelligence is taking huge steps. Generally, oncologists team up in growth sheets to talk about complex cases and figure out treatment plans. Man-made intelligence stages can work with virtual growth sheets by accumulating and examining patient information, giving proof based suggestions, and smoothing out the dynamic interaction. This cooperative methodology guarantees that patients get the aggregate mastery of a multidisciplinary group, paying little mind to geological limitations.

The execution of man-made intelligence in oncology isn't restricted to analytic and treatment perspectives; it likewise reaches out to the domain of medication disclosure. Growing new malignant growth drugs is a tedious and exorbitant interaction. Artificial intelligence speeds up this cycle by filtering through immense datasets to distinguish potential medication applicants, foresee their adequacy, and streamline treatment regimens. This holds the commitment of putting up new and inventive treatments for sale to the public all the more quickly, eventually helping malignant growth patients around the world.

Artificial intelligence's effect on persistent administration and checking is similarly significant. Distant patient checking, worked with by wearable gadgets and savvy sensors, permits persistent information assortment on essential signs, actual work, and treatment adherence.

Simulated intelligence calculations can investigate this constant information to identify early indications of treatment-related aftereffects or sickness movement, empowering convenient intercessions and acclimations to the therapy plan.

Moreover, simulated intelligence adds to the field of prognostics by anticipating patient results in light of different factors, for example, sickness stage, hereditary markers, and therapy reaction. These prescient models help oncologists in guiding patients about their anticipation, settling on informed conclusions about treatment choices, and making arrangements for long haul care.

In spite of the gigantic capability of artificial intelligence in oncology, a few difficulties and moral contemplations should be tended to. One central issue is the requirement for enormous, various datasets to successfully prepare computer based intelligence calculations. The quality and representativeness of these datasets straightforwardly influence the exhibition and generalizability of man-made intelligence models.

Guaranteeing that artificial intelligence frameworks are prepared on information that envelop different segment gatherings and sickness introductions is fundamental to keep away from predispositions and abberations in medical services results.

One more test is the interpretability of simulated intelligence calculations. As these frameworks become more complicated, understanding the reasoning behind their proposals turns out to be progressively troublesome. The "discovery" nature of some simulated intelligence models raises worries about responsibility and straight-forwardness, particularly in basic medical care choices. Endeavors to foster reasonable man-made intelligence models and lay out clear rules for their arrangement are crucial for assemble trust among medical care experts and patients.

Moral contemplations likewise emerge with regards to patient protection and infor-mation security. The broad utilization of patient information for preparing computer based intelligence models requires hearty measures to defend delicate data. Laying out rigid moral structures and administrative principles is critical to guarantee that patient security is safeguarded, and information is utilized dependably.

Moreover, there is a requirement for progressing instruction and preparing for medical services experts to adjust to the incorporation of simulated intelligence into clinical practice. Understanding how to decipher computer based intelligence pro-duced experiences, integrating these bits of knowledge into independent direction, and keeping up with compelling correspondence with patients are fundamental abili-ties that medical services suppliers should get.

Notwithstanding these difficulties, the continuous joint effort between technol-ogists, medical services experts, specialists, and policymakers is driving the quick progression of computer based intelligence in oncology.

The reconciliation of artificial intelligence into routine clinical practice can pos-sibly reshape the scene of disease care, introducing a time of customized, information driven medication.

Looking forward, the fate of computer based intelligence in oncology holds energiz-ing prospects. Proceeded with innovative work will probably prompt more complex simulated intelligence models with further developed precision and dependability. As the field advances, the cooperative energy among computer based intelligence and other arising innovations, for example, blockchain and unified learning, may addi-tionally upgrade information security, interoperability, and coordinated effort across medical services frameworks.

The democratization of man-made intelligence innovations is one more area of interest. Guaranteeing that computer based intelligence instruments are available and reasonable for medical care suppliers universally can assist with overcoming any barrier among high-and low-asset settings, eventually helping patients around the world. This inclusivity lines up with the more extensive objective of accomplishing evenhanded medical services results for all.

All in all, the reconciliation of man-made reasoning into oncology addresses a change in outlook in the manner in which we comprehend, analyze, and treat malignant growth. From early location and exact analysis to customized therapy plans and continuous checking, man-made intelligence is reshaping each part of malignant growth care. While challenges and moral contemplations persevere, continuous exploration and cooperative endeavors vow to conquer these obstacles, preparing for a future where computer based intelligence is a fundamental piece of the oncologist's tool compartment. As we forge ahead with this extraordinary excursion, a definitive objective is clear: to work on understanding results, upgrade the nature of care, and add to the worldwide battle against disease.

7.1 The role of artificial intelligence in cancer diagnosis and treatment

Man-made reasoning (artificial intelligence) has arisen as a progressive power in the domain of malignant growth finding and treatment, offering uncommon chances to improve the exactness, productivity, and personalization of medical services mediations. The multi-layered nature of malignant growth, portrayed by its hereditary variety and complex atomic profiles, makes it an optimal possibility for computer based intelligence applications. From early location to treatment arranging and progressing checking, computer based intelligence is reshaping the scene of oncology, introducing a period of accuracy medication.

In the area of disease determination, one of the most effective uses of man-made intelligence is in clinical imaging examination. Generally, the translation of radiological pictures, like X-beams, registered tomography (CT) filters, and attractive reverberation imaging (X-ray), has depended on the mastery of radiologists.

In any case, simulated intelligence calculations, especially those in light of profound learning, have shown striking capacities in picture acknowledgment and examination. These calculations can rapidly and precisely recognize examples, abnormalities, and unpretentious elements in clinical pictures, prompting early and exact malignant growth location.

The speed and effectiveness of man-made intelligence controlled picture examination are especially worthwhile with regards to disease analysis. Convenient discovery is critical for working on understanding results, as beginning phase diseases are much of the time more treatable and related with better guesses. Via mechanizing the examination of clinical pictures, man-made intelligence frameworks can speed up the ID of possible malignancies, considering brief intercession and treatment commencement.

Besides, artificial intelligence succeeds in the joining of different information hotspots for a far reaching comprehension of malignant growth. Genomic information, which gives bits of knowledge into the hereditary changes and modifications related with malignant growth, is a vital part in the period of accuracy medication. Computer based intelligence calculations can investigate tremendous genomic datasets to distinguish explicit biomarkers demonstrative of disease subtypes, guess, and potential treatment reactions. This empowers oncologists to tailor therapy plans in view of the extraordinary sub-atomic qualities of every patient's malignant growth, creating some distance from a one-size-fits-all methodology.

The idea of radiomics, which includes the extraction and investigation of quantitative elements from clinical pictures, is another region where simulated intelligence exhibits its ability. By extricating unpretentious examples and quantitative information from radiological pictures, computer based intelligence calculations can add to a more profound comprehension of growth qualities, supporting conclusion and treatment arranging. Radiomics coordinates imaging, clinical, and genomic information, giving a comprehensive perspective on the sickness that goes past what can be seen through customary imaging alone.

Notwithstanding symptomatic capacities, artificial intelligence assumes a pivotal part in treatment arranging by helping oncologists in formulating customized and designated restorative techniques. Treatment choices are many times complex, requiring thought of elements like growth qualities, patient wellbeing status, and the possible results of different mediations. Man-made intelligence calculations influence AI methods to investigate patient information, including clinical narratives, treatment reactions, and results, to suggest ideal treatment plans.

The mix of man-made intelligence in treatment arranging remains closely connected with the idea of accuracy medication. Accuracy medication intends to fit clinical intercessions to the singular qualities of every patient, streamlining the probability of treatment accomplishment while limiting antagonistic impacts.

Man-made intelligence's capacity to process and decipher tremendous datasets empowers the distinguishing proof of examples and connections that may not be evident through customary investigation techniques. This works with the determination of therapies that are probably going to be successful for a particular patient, adding to more customized and designated disease care.

In addition, simulated intelligence adds to the continuous advancement of virtual cancer sheets. Generally, cancer sheets include multidisciplinary groups of medical services experts teaming up to examine complex cases and figure out therapy plans. Simulated intelligence works with virtual growth sheets by totaling and examining patient information, giving proof based suggestions, and smoothing out the dynamic cycle. This cooperative methodology guarantees that patients benefit from the aggregate ability of trained professionals, paying little heed to geological requirements.

The field of medication revelation is another area where man-made intelligence is making critical advances in disease examination and treatment. Growing new disease drugs is a tedious and costly interaction, frequently set apart by high disappointment rates. Computer based intelligence speeds up drug revelation by filtering through huge datasets to distinguish potential medication competitors, anticipate their adequacy, and advance treatment regimens. This can possibly put up new and imaginative treatments for sale to the public all the more quickly, offering novel choices for disease patients.

Man-made intelligence's effect on persistent administration reaches out to remote observing and continuous information examination. Wearable gadgets and brilliant sensors empower consistent checking of crucial signs, actual work, and treatment adherence. Computer based intelligence calculations can break down this continuous information to distinguish early indications of treatment-related secondary effects or sickness movement, empowering convenient intercessions and changes in accordance with the therapy plan. Remote checking upgrades patient commitment, works on the nature of care, and adds to better generally results.

Prognostic demonstrating is another region where man-made intelligence gives important bits of knowledge in disease care. By utilizing AI procedures, man-made intelligence calculations can foresee patient results in light of different elements, including sickness stage, hereditary markers, and therapy reaction. These prescient models help oncologists in guiding patients about their visualization, settling on informed conclusions about treatment choices, and making arrangements for long haul care.

Notwithstanding the gigantic capability of artificial intelligence in malignant growth conclusion and treatment, a few difficulties and moral contemplations should be tended to. One of the essential difficulties is the requirement for huge, different datasets to successfully prepare computer based intelligence calculations. The quality and representativeness of these datasets straightforwardly influence the presentation and generalizability of artificial intelligence models.

Guaranteeing that man-made intelligence frameworks are prepared on information that envelop different segment gatherings and illness introductions is fundamental to stay away from predispositions and abberations in medical care results.

The interpretability of computer based intelligence calculations is another test that requires cautious thought. As man-made intelligence models become more mind boggling, understanding the reasoning behind their proposals turns out to be progressively troublesome. The "discovery" nature of some computer based intelligence models raises worries about responsibility and straightforwardness, particularly in basic medical care choices. Endeavors to foster reasonable simulated intelligence models and lay out clear rules for their sending are significant to assemble trust among medical services experts and patients.

Moral contemplations likewise emerge with regards to patient protection and information security. The broad utilization of patient information for preparing man-made intelligence models requires strong measures to shield delicate data. Laying out rigid moral systems and administrative guidelines is fundamental to guarantee that patient security is safeguarded, and information is utilized mindfully.

Besides, there is a requirement for continuous schooling and preparing for medical services experts to adjust to the combination of computer based intelligence into clinical practice. Understanding how to decipher artificial intelligence created experiences, integrating these bits of knowledge into direction, and keeping up with successful correspondence with patients are fundamental abilities that medical services suppliers should secure.

Regardless of these difficulties, the continuous coordinated effort between technologists, medical care experts, scientists, and policymakers is driving the fast headway of simulated intelligence in malignant growth finding and therapy. The mix of man-made intelligence into routine clinical practice can possibly reshape the scene of malignant growth care, introducing a period of customized, information driven medication.

Looking forward, the eventual fate of computer based intelligence in disease finding and treatment holds energizing prospects. Proceeded with innovative work will probably prompt more refined artificial intelligence models with further developed precision and dependability. As the field develops, the cooperative energy among simulated intelligence and other arising advancements, for example, blockchain and unified learning, may additionally improve information security, interoperability, and coordinated effort across medical care frameworks.

The democratization of man-made intelligence innovations is one more area of interest. Guaranteeing that man-made intelligence apparatuses are available and reasonable for medical care suppliers internationally can assist with overcoming any issues among high-and low-asset settings, at last helping patients around the world. This inclusivity lines up with the more extensive objective of accomplishing even-handed medical services results for all.

All in all, the job of man-made reasoning in malignant growth determination and therapy is extraordinary, offering exceptional chances to change the manner in which we get it, recognize, and oversee disease. From early recognition through clinical imaging examination to customized treatment arranging and progressing observing, simulated intelligence is an incredible asset in the possession of medical care experts. While challenges and moral contemplations continue, progressing research and co-operative endeavors vow to defeat these obstacles, preparing for a future where man-made intelligence is an essential and basic piece of the oncologist's tool compartment. As we forge ahead with this extraordinary excursion, a definitive objective is clear: to work on persistent results, improve the nature of care, and add to the worldwide battle against malignant growth.

7.2 Machine learning algorithms for predicting treatment outcomes

AI (ML) calculations have arisen as integral assets in medical care, offering the possibility to change therapy results by utilizing prescient demonstrating and infor-mation driven bits of knowledge. With regards to foreseeing treatment results, ML calculations assume a pivotal part in dissecting different datasets, recognizing designs, and creating expectations that help medical services experts in settling on informed choices. This utilization of ML is especially huge in oncology, where the intricacy of malignant growth and the changeability of treatment reactions require customized and exact methodologies.

One of the essential utilizations of ML in anticipating therapy results is in the field of disease treatment. The capacity to foresee how a singular patient will answer a particular treatment is priceless in fitting mediations to boost viability and limit unfriendly impacts. ML calculations use various information sources, including patient socioeconomics, clinical history, hereditary data, and treatment reaction information, to foster prescient models.

The idea of accuracy medication is firmly lined up with the objectives of anticipating treatment results utilizing ML. Accuracy medication means to fit clinical mediations to the singular qualities of every patient, perceiving that varieties in hereditary cosmetics, way of life, and natural elements add to contrasts in treatment reactions. ML calculations succeed in taking care of the intricacy of these datasets and distinguishing applicable examples that can illuminate customized treatment plans.

In the domain of disease treatment, ML calculations add to treatment determination by examining authentic patient information and results related with explicit treatments. This empowers the distinguishing proof of examples that associate with positive reactions or protection from specific medicines. By taking into account a huge number of variables, including hereditary markers, growth qualities, and patient socioeconomics, ML models can produce expectations about the probability of progress for various treatment choices.

Besides, ML calculations assume a crucial part in foreseeing and overseeing treatment-related secondary effects. These calculations investigate patient information to distinguish risk factors related with unfavorable responses to explicit medicines. By anticipating the probability of aftereffects, medical care suppliers can proactively execute measures to relieve these impacts or change therapy designs appropriately. This proactive methodology upgrades patient security and adds to the general nature of care.

In the domain of ongoing sicknesses, for example, diabetes and cardiovascular circumstances, ML calculations are utilized to anticipate therapy results by dissecting patient information after some time. These calculations can consider different boundaries, including blood glucose levels, way of life variables, and medicine adherence, to figure infection movement and designer treatment plans. This prescient demonstrating works with early intercession and customized acclimations to treatment systems, at last working on persistent results.

Besides, ML calculations add to anticipating treatment reactions in irresistible illnesses, like viral contaminations and bacterial sicknesses. For instance, with regards to antiretroviral treatment for HIV, ML models can break down quiet information to anticipate virologic reactions and guide the determination of ideal medication regimens. Essentially, in the field of anti-toxin treatment, ML calculations influence information on microbial obstruction examples and patient elements to foresee the adequacy of various anti-toxin decisions.

The prescient force of ML isn't restricted to treatment viability; it additionally stretches out to the expectation of illness repeat. In oncology, foreseeing the probability of malignant growth repeat after treatment is a basic part of long haul the board. ML calculations break down a mix of clinical, imaging, and genomic information to foster models that can gauge the gamble of repeat for individual patients. These expectations illuminate choices about post-therapy observation techniques and the power of follow-up care.

The coordination of ML calculations in foreseeing treatment results requires the accessibility of huge and various datasets. The quality and representativeness of these datasets straightforwardly influence the presentation and generalizability of ML models. Consequently, endeavors to guarantee information inclusivity and address likely predispositions in datasets are fundamental to foster hearty and solid prescient models.

Interpretable and reasonable man-made intelligence models are significant in medical care, particularly while anticipating therapy results. The capacity to comprehend the reasoning behind expectations is fundamental for acquiring trust among medical care experts and patients. Endeavors to improve the interpretability of ML models, like creating straightforward calculations and giving clear clarifications to expectations, add to the moral sending of these advancements in clinical practice.

Regardless of the commitments and potential, the use of ML in foreseeing treatment results isn't without challenges. One critical test is the requirement for constant model approval and refinement. Medical care information is dynamic, and therapy rehearses advance after some time. ML models should be consistently refreshed to integrate new information and guarantee their proceeded with exactness and significance.

Besides, the generalizability of ML models across different patient populaces and medical services settings is a worry. Models prepared on information from one populace may not perform ideally when applied to an alternate segment or geographic locale. Guaranteeing the strength and appropriateness of ML models in different settings is fundamental for their broad reception and effect on treatment results.

Another test is the moral utilization of prescient models in medical care. The potential for predisposition in calculations, especially when prepared on imbalanced or fragmented datasets, raises worries about fair admittance to precise expectations. Tending to these predispositions and guaranteeing that ML models don't propagate or worsen existing medical services variations is a basic thought in the mindful sending of these advances.

Notwithstanding challenges, moral contemplations additionally stretch out to issues of patient protection and information security. ML calculations depend on immense measures of delicate patient information for preparing and approval. Laying out rigid security shields and adherence to administrative norms is basic to safeguard patient secrecy and keep up with public confidence in the utilization of man-made intelligence for anticipating treatment results.

Notwithstanding these difficulties and moral contemplations, the continuous advancement in the field of ML for anticipating treatment results holds massive commitment. The coordinated effort between medical services experts, analysts, information researchers, and policymakers is fundamental to explore these difficulties and open the maximum capacity of ML in customized and exact medication.

Looking forward, the eventual fate of ML in foreseeing treatment results includes headways in algorithmic refinement, expanded cooperation, and a promise to tending to moral contemplations. As innovation keeps on developing, the incorporation of ML into routine clinical practice can possibly upset treatment direction, work on persistent results, and add to a more customized and viable way to deal with medical services. The excursion towards utilizing ML for anticipating treatment results is a continuous and dynamic cycle, with a definitive objective of improving the nature of care and propelling the field of medication into another period of information driven accuracy.

7.3 Examples of AI applications in cancer research and treatment

Computerized reasoning (computer based intelligence) applications in disease exploration and treatment have multiplied as of late, displaying the groundbreaking capability of these advancements in further developing results, speeding up research, and customizing patient consideration. Across different phases of disease care, from early discovery to treatment arranging and checking, simulated intelligence is making huge commitments. Looking at explicit models shows the different and effective manners by which man-made intelligence is reshaping the scene of malignant growth examination and treatment.

In the domain of malignant growth diagnostics, computer based intelligence has shown astounding abilities in breaking down clinical pictures for early location. One eminent model is the use of computer based intelligence in bosom malignant growth screening utilizing mammography. Conventional mammogram translation can be testing and is dependent upon human blunder. Man-made intelligence calculations, especially those in light of profound learning, have shown guarantee in upgrading the precision of mammogram readings.

These calculations can break down mammographic pictures to distinguish unpretentious examples and inconsistencies characteristic of beginning phase bosom disease. Via preparing on huge datasets with explained pictures, simulated intelligence models can figure out how to perceive irregularities that might be ignored by human spectators. The outcome is a more exact and convenient recognition of bosom malignant growth, possibly prompting prior mediation and further developed results for patients.

Notwithstanding mammography, man-made intelligence is gaining ground in the examination of other clinical imaging modalities, like processed tomography (CT) and attractive reverberation imaging (X-ray). For instance, in cellular breakdown in the lungs analysis, simulated intelligence calculations can aid the recognizable proof and portrayal of pneumonic knobs. Early recognition of lung knobs is essential for opportune finding and mediation, and simulated intelligence's capacity to handle enormous volumes of imaging information upgrades the proficiency of radiologists in distinguishing possible malignancies.

Additionally, man-made intelligence applications stretch out past picture examination to pathology. Pathologists assume a critical part in malignant growth finding by looking at tissue tests to recognize the presence of disease cells and decide their qualities. Computer based intelligence fueled pathology apparatuses can help pathologists via mechanizing specific undertakings, for example, distinguishing districts of interest in pathology slides or supporting the arrangement of various cell types. This cooperative methodology among man-made intelligence and pathologists can possibly smooth out the analytic cycle, decrease responsibility, and upgrade demonstrative precision.

Genomic investigation is another region where computer based intelligence is altering disease exploration and treatment. The genomic intricacy of malignant growth, described by different transformations and adjustments, presents difficulties in recognizing significant bits of knowledge. Simulated intelligence calculations can filter through immense genomic datasets to recognize examples and affiliations that may not be evident through customary examination strategies.

For example, in the ID of malignant growth biomarkers, simulated intelligence can dissect genomic information to pinpoint explicit hereditary marks related with various disease types or treatment reactions. These biomarkers act as important pointers for fitting treatment techniques to individual patients, adding to the worldview of accuracy medication. In colorectal disease, for instance, man-made intelligence driven genomic examination can recognize explicit changes that impact guess and guide treatment choices.

Therapy arranging is a basic stage in malignant growth care, and man-made intelligence is progressively assuming a part in streamlining remedial methodologies. One eminent model is the utilization of man-made intelligence in radiation treatment arranging. Radiation treatment includes exactly focusing on malignant growth cells with remedial radiation while saving encompassing sound tissues. Artificial intelligence calculations can examine patient life structures, growth attributes, and therapy objectives to advance radiation therapy plans.

By utilizing AI, these calculations can produce designs that accomplish remedial objectives with decreased radiation openness to sound tissues. This works on the adequacy of radiation treatment as well as limits secondary effects for patients. The reconciliation of computer based intelligence in radiation treatment arranging epitomizes how innovation can upgrade therapy accuracy and individualize remedial mediations.

With regards to chemotherapy, simulated intelligence applications add to advancing medication choice and dosing. Chemotherapy regimens are frequently connected with aftereffects, and fitting medicines to individual patient profiles can further develop results and decrease antagonistic impacts. Man-made intelligence calculations can investigate patient information, including hereditary data, treatment history, and reaction designs, to anticipate ideal chemotherapy regimens for explicit people.

Besides, computer based intelligence upholds drug revelation and advancement, tending to the requirement for novel and designated disease treatments. Conventional medication revelation is a tedious and costly interaction, with high weakening rates. Man-made intelligence speeds up this cycle by investigating huge datasets, including atomic and clinical information, to recognize potential medication applicants and foresee their viability.

For example, in distinguishing drug mixes with synergistic impacts, artificial intelligence models can dissect the collaborations between various mixtures and anticipate blends that improve helpful results. This approach holds guarantee for conquering obstruction instruments and working on the viability of disease medicines.

Clinical preliminary matching is another computer based intelligence application that smoothes out the most common way of interfacing qualified patients with fitting clinical preliminaries. Coordinating patients with applicable preliminaries is vital for propelling exploration and giving admittance to state of the art treatments. Simulated intelligence calculations can examine patient information, including clinical profiles and genomic data, to distinguish reasonable clinical preliminary open doors.

This customized way to deal with clinical preliminary coordinating guarantees that patients are associated with preliminaries that line up with their singular qualities, improving the probability of effective enlistment. The mix of artificial intelligence in clinical preliminary matching adds to the productivity of preliminary enlistment and speeds up the advancement of new malignant growth medicines.

Far off understanding observing is an arising simulated intelligence application that upgrades post-treatment care and long haul the executives. Wearable gadgets and sensors furnished with man-made intelligence calculations empower nonstop checking of patients' important bodily functions, active work, and treatment adherence. This ongoing information permits medical services suppliers to follow patients' prosperity and identify early indications of likely issues.

With regards to malignant growth survivorship, remote checking can work with continuous observation for repeat or treatment-related incidental effects. Man-made intelligence calculations break down the gathered information to give experiences into patients' wellbeing status, empowering convenient mediations and customized care plans. This proactive way to deal with patient administration adds to worked on personal satisfaction for malignant growth survivors.

Notwithstanding the previously mentioned applications, man-made intelligence is additionally making advances into steady consideration for malignant growth patients. Normal Language Handling (NLP) calculations, a subset of man-made intelligence, are utilized to investigate printed information from electronic wellbeing records, patient gatherings, and online entertainment to acquire bits of knowledge into patients' encounters, concerns, and inclinations.

This data can educate the advancement regarding steady consideration mediations custom-made to the remarkable necessities of individual patients. For example, feeling examination of patient accounts can distinguish profound prosperity patterns, and man-made intelligence driven chatbots or menial helpers can offer customized help and data to patients all through their malignant growth venture.

Regardless of the various advantages and promising applications, the reconciliation of artificial intelligence in malignant growth exploration and treatment isn't without challenges. One critical test is the requirement for huge, different, and great datasets for preparing artificial intelligence calculations really. The exhibition and generalizability of man-made intelligence models rely upon the representativeness of the information they are prepared on. Endeavors to guarantee inclusivity and address predispositions in datasets are fundamental for the capable turn of events and organization of simulated intelligence applications in disease care.

Interpretability of artificial intelligence models is another test that requires consideration. As artificial intelligence calculations become more mind boggling, understanding the thinking behind their expectations turns out to be progressively troublesome. The absence of interpretability raises worries about the responsibility and straightforwardness of man-made intelligence driven choices, particularly in basic medical services settings. Endeavors to foster logical computer based intelligence models and lay out clear rules for their organization are crucial for fabricate trust among medical care experts and patients.

Moral contemplations likewise emerge concerning patient protection and information security. The broad utilization of patient information for preparing and approval purposes requires powerful measures to protect delicate data. Laying out severe moral structures and administrative guidelines is basic to guarantee patient security is safeguarded, and information is utilized dependably.

Also, the joining of simulated intelligence advances into routine clinical practice requires progressing instruction and preparing for medical services experts. Understanding how to decipher artificial intelligence created experiences, integrating these bits of knowledge into direction, and keeping up with compelling correspondence with patients are fundamental abilities that medical services suppliers should procure to completely use the capability of simulated intelligence in malignant growth care.

Disease exploration and treatment have gone through critical changes with the mix of trend setting innovations, especially Computerized reasoning (artificial intelligence). The multi-layered nature of disease, portrayed by its hereditary variety and complex sub-atomic profiles, makes it an optimal contender for imaginative methodologies that influence simulated intelligence to further develop results, customize treatment, and speed up research endeavors.

One of the key regions where simulated intelligence has exhibited significant effect is in early disease recognition through cutting edge imaging examination. Mammography, a critical device in bosom malignant growth screening, has seen upgrades in precision and productivity with the guide of computer based intelligence calculations.

Profound learning models, prepared on huge datasets of mammographic pictures, can perceive unpretentious examples and oddities demonstrative of beginning phase bosom disease. The utilization of man-made intelligence in mammography upgrades the responsiveness of screenings, empowering prior identification and mediation, eventually adding to worked on quiet results.

Past mammography, artificial intelligence is taking critical steps in the examination of other clinical imaging modalities. For example, in cellular breakdown in the lungs conclusion, man-made intelligence calculations can aid the ID and portrayal of aspiratory knobs through the examination of processed tomography (CT) filters. The capacity of man-made intelligence to handle huge volumes of imaging information improves the speed and precision of recognizing expected malignancies, giving a significant instrument to early location and finding.

Pathology, a basic part of malignant growth determination, has likewise profited from simulated intelligence applications. Pathologists generally investigate tissue tests to distinguish disease cells and decide their attributes. Artificial intelligence controlled pathology devices mechanize specific undertakings, supporting pathologists in the translation of pathology slides. This cooperation among simulated intelligence and pathologists smoothes out the analytic interaction, lessens responsibility, and improves the precision of disease analyze.

Genomic examination, one more foundation of disease research, has seen an upset with the use of simulated intelligence. The perplexing and tremendous datasets created through genomic profiling are appropriate for computer based intelligence calculations. These calculations can distinguish examples and relationship inside genomic information, revealing hereditary markers and changes related with explicit disease types or treatment reactions. Artificial intelligence driven genomic investigation adds to the improvement of designated treatments and the acknowledgment of accuracy medication, where therapies are customized to the singular attributes of every patient's disease.

Therapy arranging, a critical part of disease care, has been upset by man-made intelligence, especially in radiation treatment. Man-made intelligence calculations examine patient life systems, growth qualities, and therapy objectives to streamline radiation therapy plans. By utilizing AI, these calculations create plans that accomplish helpful objectives with decreased radiation openness to solid tissues. This works on the viability of radiation treatment as well as limits secondary effects for patients, featuring the potential for artificial intelligence to upgrade therapy accuracy.

Chemotherapy, a foundation of disease treatment, benefits from computer based intelligence applications in streamlining drug determination and dosing. Computer based intelligence calculations investigate patient information, including hereditary data, treatment history, and reaction designs, to anticipate ideal chemotherapy regimens for explicit people.

This customized way to deal with chemotherapy limits unfavorable impacts and further develops treatment results by fitting mediations to individual patient profiles.

In the domain of medication revelation and advancement, simulated intelligence speeds up the ID of potential medication competitors and the streamlining of treatment regimens. The customary medication disclosure process is tedious and expensive, with high disappointment rates. Simulated intelligence, by investigating tremendous datasets including atomic and clinical information, predicts the adequacy of medication applicants, possibly smoothing out the advancement of new malignant growth treatments. The capacity of simulated intelligence to distinguish synergistic impacts between various mixtures holds guarantee for conquering obstruction components and working on the adequacy of disease medicines.

Clinical preliminary coordinating, a basic part of propelling disease research, is likewise worked with by man-made intelligence applications. These calculations dissect patient information, including clinical profiles and genomic data, to distinguish reasonable clinical preliminary open doors. By coordinating patients with significant preliminaries in light of their singular attributes, simulated intelligence smoothes out the enrollment cycle, guaranteeing that patients are associated with preliminaries that line up with their remarkable profiles. This customized way to deal with clinical preliminary matching adds to the effectiveness of preliminary enlistment and speeds up the advancement of new malignant growth medicines.

Distant patient observing, an arising field in malignant growth care, uses wearable gadgets and sensors furnished with computer based intelligence calculations to empower constant checking of patients' important bodily functions, actual work, and treatment adherence. This ongoing information permits medical services suppliers to follow patients' prosperity and recognize early indications of expected issues. With regards to malignant growth survivorship, remote checking works with progressing observation for repeat or treatment-related secondary effects. Man-made intelligence driven investigation of gathered information gives experiences into patients' wellbeing status, empowering convenient mediations and customized care plans.

Strong consideration for disease patients has additionally seen the combination of simulated intelligence applications. Regular Language Handling (NLP) calculations, a subset of computer based intelligence, investigate text based information from electronic wellbeing records, patient discussions, and virtual entertainment to acquire bits of knowledge into patients' encounters, concerns, and inclinations. This data illuminates the advancement regarding steady consideration intercessions custom fitted to the one of a kind requirements of individual patients. Opinion investigation of patient stories, for instance, can distinguish close to home prosperity patterns, and computer based intelligence driven chatbots or remote helpers can offer customized help and data to patients all through their malignant growth venture.

In spite of the bunch benefits and promising applications, the joining of artificial intelligence in malignant growth examination and treatment isn't without challenges. One critical test is the requirement for enormous, different, and top notch datasets for preparing artificial intelligence calculations successfully. The exhibition and generalizability of simulated intelligence models rely upon the representativeness of the information they are prepared on. Endeavors to guarantee inclusivity and address predispositions in datasets are fundamental for the capable turn of events and organization of man-made intelligence applications in disease care.

Interpretability of simulated intelligence models is another test that requires consideration. As simulated intelligence calculations become more intricate, understanding the thinking behind their expectations turns out to be progressively troublesome. The absence of interpretability raises worries about the responsibility and straightforwardness of artificial intelligence driven choices, particularly in basic medical services settings. Endeavors to foster reasonable simulated intelligence models and lay out clear rules for their organization are fundamental for construct trust among medical care experts and patients.

Moral contemplations additionally emerge concerning patient protection and information security. The broad utilization of patient information for preparing and approval purposes requires strong measures to protect delicate data. Laying out severe moral systems and administrative principles is basic to guarantee patient security is safeguarded, and information is utilized mindfully.

Moreover, the coordination of computer based intelligence innovations into routine clinical practice requires continuous instruction and preparing for medical care experts. Understanding how to decipher artificial intelligence produced bits of knowledge, integrating these experiences into navigation, and keeping up with successful correspondence with patients are fundamental abilities that medical services suppliers should gain to completely use the capability of computer based intelligence in disease care.

All in all, the instances of computer based intelligence applications in malignant growth exploration and therapy feature the extraordinary effect of these advances on different parts of disease care. From early location and conclusion to therapy arranging, drug revelation, and strong consideration, artificial intelligence is reshaping the scene of disease examination and treatment. As innovation keeps on developing, the joining of computer based intelligence into routine clinical practice can possibly upset treatment navigation, work on quiet results, and add to a more customized and compelling way to deal with medical care. The continuous advancement in this field highlights the significance of cooperative endeavors among medical services experts, analysts, information researchers, and policymakers to explore difficulties, guarantee moral use, and open the maximum capacity of simulated intelligence in propelling malignant growth care.

Chapter 8

Patient-Centered Approaches

Patient-focused approaches in medical services have earned expanding respect as fundamental components in conveying superior grade, empathetic, and powerful clinical consideration. The shift towards patient-focused care implies a takeoff from conventional models that frequently focus on illness driven viewpoints and supplier driven navigation. All things being equal, patient-focused approaches focus on the singular's novel necessities, values, and inclinations, encouraging a cooperative and comprehensive medical care climate.

At the center of patient-focused care is the affirmation that patients are specialists in their own lives. This acknowledgment urges medical services experts to draw in patients effectively in their consideration, advancing shared direction and fitting therapy intends to line up with the patient's objectives and inclinations. Fundamentally, patient-focused care is a worldview that puts the patient at the focal point of the medical services insight, advancing a comprehensive comprehension of wellbeing that reaches out past the simple shortfall of sickness.

One critical part of patient-focused approaches includes successful correspondence between medical care suppliers and patients. Correspondence is the key part that associates clinical mastery with the patient's experiential information. Open and straightforward correspondence constructs trust, improves understanding, and enables patients to take part in choices about their wellbeing effectively. Successful correspondence likewise includes undivided attention, recognizing patients' interests, and answering compassionately to their necessities.

Notwithstanding correspondence, shared independent direction is a basic part of patient-focused care. This cooperative cycle includes medical services suppliers and patients cooperating to arrive at conclusions about the patient's consideration. Shared direction perceives that patients bring important bits of knowledge into their own inclinations, values, and ways of life, which can essentially affect the progress of treatment plans. Through shared navigation, patients become dynamic accomplices in their medical services venture, adding to a more customized and successful consideration experience.

Moreover, patient-focused care stretches out past individual connections to include the general medical services framework. It includes a pledge to social capability, perceiving and regarding the variety of patients concerning their experiences, convictions, and values. Medical services associations that embrace patient-focused approaches effectively try to kill wellbeing differences and elevate value in admittance to mind.

The execution of patient-focused care requires a foundational shift in the way of life of medical services conveyance. This change includes changes in arrangements, techniques, and the general outlook of medical care suppliers and associations. Embracing patient-focused approaches frequently requires a takeoff from the conventional paternalistic model of medical care towards a model that values coordinated effort, regard, and inclusivity.

In commonsense terms, patient-focused care includes fitting clinical medicines to the one of a kind requirements and inclinations of individual patients. This might incorporate thinking about a patient's social foundation, financial status, and individual convictions while fostering a consideration plan. In doing as such, medical care suppliers can make more powerful and patient-accommodating mediations that reverberate with the singular's way of life and values.

The idea of patient-focused care additionally perceives the significance of tending to the actual parts of wellbeing as well as the close to home, social, and mental aspects. This comprehensive methodology thinks about the effect of disease on a patient's general prosperity and personal satisfaction. Thus, patient-focused care might include incorporating psychosocial support, psychological wellness administrations, and assets for patients and their families.

Patient-focused care is especially important in ongoing illness the board, where long haul commitment and joint effort among patients and medical services suppliers are vital. Persistent circumstances frequently require continuous self-administration, and patients assume a focal

part in coming to conclusions about their consideration on an everyday premise. In such cases, patient-focused approaches enable people to become dynamic members in their wellbeing the executives, encouraging a feeling of independence and control.

The advantages of patient-focused care reach out past the singular patient to the medical services framework overall. Studies have shown that patient-focused approaches add to worked on understanding fulfillment, adherence to treatment plans, and wellbeing results. By including patients in their consideration, medical services suppliers can likewise improve productivity and decrease medical services costs by keeping away from pointless mediations and hospitalizations.

Notwithstanding the various benefits of patient-focused care, its far reaching reception faces difficulties inside the ongoing medical services scene. One huge obstruction is the dug in custom of the various leveled supplier patient relationship, where the medical services proficient is much of the time apparent as the sole power. Moving towards a more cooperative model requires a social change that difficulties existing power elements and advances a mutual perspective of mastery.

Another test includes time requirements inside medical care settings. The customary model of care frequently focuses on productivity, with restricted time for patient cooperations. Carrying out quiet focused care requires assigning adequate time for significant discussions, undivided attention, and shared independent direction. This requires a reexamination of medical services conveyance models and asset portion to help these fundamental parts of patient-focused care.

The mix of innovation into medical care presents the two open doors and difficulties for patient-focused approaches. On one hand, innovation can upgrade correspondence, work with remote observing, and give patients significant wellbeing data. Then again, the rising dependence on electronic wellbeing records and mechanized frameworks may coincidentally depersonalize the patient-supplier relationship. Finding some kind of harmony among innovation and human-focused care is critical for the fruitful execution of patient-focused approaches.

Schooling and preparing are critical in encouraging a medical services labor force that embraces patient-focused care. Medical care experts need to foster abilities in viable correspondence, social capability, and shared direction. Moreover, ingraining a patient-focused mentality requires progressing schooling to stay up with developing medical care rehearses and the coordination of new proof based approaches.

The patient's viewpoint on their medical services experience is a key measurement in assessing the progress of patient-focused care. Patient-announced results (Aces) give significant bits of knowledge into the effect of sickness and therapy on the patient's personal satisfaction. These results can advise medical care suppliers about the viability regarding mediations and guide changes in accordance with therapy plans in view of the patient's insight.

Patient-focused approaches are especially important with regards to preventive consideration and wellbeing advancement. Engaging people to play a functioning job in keeping up with their wellbeing can add to the avoidance of illnesses and the advancement of in general prosperity. This proactive methodology includes teaching patients about solid way of life decisions, preventive screenings, and early identification of potential medical problems.

The idea of patient-focused care lines up with the standards of individual focused medication, which stresses the significance of grasping patients as one of a kind people with their own stories, values, and objectives. Individual focused medication rises above the reductionist methodology that sees patients exclusively from the perspective of their illnesses. All things considered, it perceives the interconnectedness of physical, mental, and social elements in forming a singular's wellbeing.

Firmly connected with individual focused medication is the idea of account medication, which highlights the meaning of narrating in medical care. Perceiving that disease isn't just an organic peculiarity yet in addition a story experience, story medication urges medical care suppliers to stand by listening to patients' accounts, grasp their points of view, and coordinate these accounts into the more extensive setting of care.

The reception of patient-focused care isn't restricted to explicit clinical claims to fame yet is material across many disciplines. Whether in essential consideration, specialty facilities, or medical clinic settings, patient-focused approaches upgrade the general nature of care and add to positive patient encounters. This inclusivity builds up the possibility that patient-focused care is a major part of medical services conveyance instead of a specific practice.

Patient commitment is a focal precept of patient-focused care, stressing the dynamic contribution of people in their medical services venture. Connected with patients are bound to stick to treatment plans, partake in shared navigation, and take responsibility for wellbeing. Medical care suppliers can work with patient commitment by encouraging a cooperative and engaging climate that esteems the info and viewpoints of people.

The idea of patient-focused care stretches out past the clinical setting to envelop the more extensive medical services environment, including wellbeing strategy and support. Support for patient-focused approaches includes perceiving patients as partners in medical services navigation and guaranteeing their portrayal in conversations about medical services conveyance, exploration, and asset distribution. Strategies that focus on quiet focused approaches add to a more responsive and fair medical services framework.

8.1 Importance of considering the patient's perspective in cancer treatment

The significance of considering the patient's point of view in disease treatment couldn't possibly be more significant, as it significantly impacts the general insight, prosperity, and results for people confronting this difficult analysis. Disease, a complex and frequently life changing condition, requires an exhaustive methodology that goes past clinical intercessions to incorporate the profound, mental, and social elements of the patient's excursion.

From the snapshot of conclusion, patients set out on a wild and unsure way. Understanding the one of a kind difficulties and fears that every individual countenances is significant in fitting malignant growth treatment intends to line up with their qualities and inclinations. The patient's point of view offers significant bits of knowledge into their objectives, needs, and assumptions, directing medical services experts in giving customized and patient-focused care.

One of the focal parts of considering the patient's point of view in malignant growth therapy is recognizing the close to home effect of a disease determination. Disease isn't simply an actual sickness; it has significant mental and close to home ramifications for the individual and their friends and family. Nervousness, dread, melancholy, and vulnerability frequently go with a malignant growth finding, and perceiving and addressing these feelings is necessary to giving all encompassing consideration.

Medical care suppliers should make an open and strong space for patients to communicate their feelings and concerns. Compelling correspondence assumes a critical part in this cycle, as it lays out a groundwork of trust and permits patients to feel appreciated and comprehended. Finding opportunity to listen effectively, approve feelings, and offer sympathetic help can altogether add to the patient's general prosperity.

Additionally, understanding the patient's point of view in malignant growth treatment includes perceiving the different ways people adapt to their analysis. Every individual brings a special arrangement of survival strategies, flexibility, and emotionally supportive networks to their disease process. Some might look for data and effectively take part in direction, while others might favor a more detached job, depending in their medical services group for direction. Fitting correspondence and inclusion methodologies in view of individual inclinations is vital to encouraging a cooperative and engaging patient-supplier relationship.

Shared navigation turns into a pivotal part of disease treatment while thinking about the patient's viewpoint. Including patients in choices about their consideration regards their independence as well as guarantees that treatment plans line up with their qualities and objectives. This cooperative methodology recognizes that patients are specialists in their own lives and energizes a feeling of organization, which can decidedly influence adherence to treatment and in general fulfillment with care.

Moreover, the patient's point of view in malignant growth therapy reaches out past clinical choices to envelop parts of day to day existence that might be impacted by the sickness and its therapy. Thought should be given to the patient's way of life, obligations, and individual objectives. This comprehensive methodology empowers medical services suppliers to tailor therapy designs that are successful in tending to the illness as well as viable with the patient's life conditions.

The effect of disease on the patient's social encouraging group of people is one more critical viewpoint to consider. Family, companions, and local area assume huge parts in offering profound help, help with reasonable issues, and a feeling of association during the difficult excursion of disease treatment. Perceiving and utilizing these emotionally supportive networks can emphatically impact the patient's insight and add to their general prosperity.

Social capability is a fundamental component in figuring out the patient's viewpoint in malignant growth treatment. People from assorted social foundations might have extraordinary convictions, values, and inclinations with respect to wellbeing and sickness. Medical services suppliers should be sensitive to social subtleties to guarantee that the consideration they convey is aware, comprehensive, and lined up with the patient's social setting. This approach encourages trust and works with compelling correspondence, eventually improving the nature of care.

Besides, taking into account the patient's viewpoint includes tending to the monetary ramifications of disease treatment. The expense of disease care, including clinical costs, meds, and strong administrations, can represent a critical weight on patients and their families. Medical services suppliers ought to be sensitive to the monetary worries of patients, offering backing, assets, and, while conceivable, talking about potential monetary ramifications forthright to help with informed navigation.

The patient's viewpoint in malignant growth treatment isn't static; it advances all through the direction of the sickness. From the underlying shock of analysis to the difficulties of treatment, survivorship, or end-of-life care, patients might encounter fluctuating feelings and requirements. Medical care suppliers should remain receptive to these changes, constantly evaluating and adjusting their way to deal with line up with the developing necessities and needs of the patient.

In the domain of disease treatment, the patient's point of view is instrumental in forming survivorship plans. Survivorship care includes tending to the physical, close to home, and social parts of life after malignant growth treatment. Understanding the patient's objectives for survivorship, whether they connect with getting back to work, revamping connections, or seeking after new life needs, illuminates the improvement regarding custom-made survivorship care designs that help the person in recovering a feeling of predictability and prosperity.

Significantly, the patient's point of view reaches out to the thought of palliative and end-of-life care with regards to cutting edge or terminal malignant growth. Transparent correspondence about forecast, treatment choices, and objectives of care is fundamental during these difficult times. Figuring out the patient's qualities, inclinations for side effect the board, and wanted personal satisfaction guides medical services suppliers in conveying humane and patient-focused finish of-life care.

Additionally, including patients ahead of time care arranging guarantees that their desires in regards to clinical mediations, revival inclinations, and other basic choices are regarded. This approach maintains the patient's independence as well as gives a structure to relatives and medical services suppliers to explore complex choices in arrangement with the patient's qualities.

The patient's point of view in disease therapy isn't just essential for individual consideration yet additionally adds to headways in malignant growth exploration and medical care strategy. Patient-revealed results (Professionals) give significant information on the effect of malignant growth and its treatment on the patient's personal satisfaction. This data helps analysts and policymakers in grasping this present reality encounters of people with disease, directing the improvement of mediations and strategies that better location patient necessities.

Besides, patient backing assumes a critical part in molding the scene of disease care. Patients and their supporters frequently add to explore, take part in clinical preliminaries, and backer for strategies that focus on understanding focused approaches. By enhancing the patient's voice in dynamic cycles, these promoters add to a more comprehensive, responsive, and patient-focused medical services framework.

All in all, the significance of considering the patient's point of view in disease treatment couldn't possibly be more significant. A diverse methodology includes perceiving the profound and mental components of the patient's excursion, fitting therapy plans to individual inclinations, taking part in shared direction, and tending to the more extensive effect of disease on the patient's life. By focusing on the patient's point of view, medical services suppliers can convey more merciful, customized, and compelling disease care, eventually working on the general insight and results for people confronting this considerable test.

8.2 Integrating holistic care and supportive therapies

The mix of all encompassing consideration and strong treatments into regular clinical methodologies is earning expanding respect as an exhaustive and patient-focused model for tending to the perplexing necessities of people confronting different wellbeing challenges. Comprehensive consideration goes past treating explicit side effects or illnesses; it thinks about the entire individual — body, brain, and soul — chasing ideal wellbeing and prosperity.

Strong treatments supplement conventional clinical intercessions by tending to the physical, close to home, and social parts of wellbeing, encouraging a more all encompassing and patient-focused way to deal with care.

All encompassing consideration accentuates the interconnectedness of various parts of a singular's wellbeing. It perceives that actual wellbeing is complicatedly connected to profound and otherworldly prosperity, and that addressing these aspects altogether can prompt more successful and manageable wellbeing results. This approach requires a shift from the reductionist perspective on medical care, which frequently centers exclusively around treating segregated side effects or sicknesses, to a more integrative and individual focused model.

Integral to all encompassing consideration is the acknowledgment of the person's intrinsic capacity to mend. The body has an exceptional limit with respect to self-guideline and recuperation, and all encompassing consideration tries to help and upgrade these normal mending processes. This point of view urges medical services suppliers to work cooperatively with patients, enabling them to play a functioning job in their wellbeing and prosperity. It includes training, direction, and shared decision-production to make an organization that regards the uniqueness of every person.

Mind-body intercessions are vital parts of all encompassing consideration, accentuating the interconnectedness of mental and actual wellbeing. Practices like care contemplation, yoga, and unwinding procedures have been displayed to decidedly affect pressure decrease, invulnerable capability, and generally prosperity. Incorporating these practices into medical services tends to the mental parts of wellbeing as well as adds to the counteraction and the executives of different states of being.

Nourishment is a major mainstay of comprehensive consideration, perceiving the significant effect of diet on generally speaking wellbeing. Dietary decisions assume a vital part in forestalling and overseeing ongoing circumstances, supporting the safe framework, and advancing ideal working of the body. Comprehensive consideration underscores customized nourishment designs that think about individual inclinations, social foundations, and wellbeing objectives. This approach goes past the one-size-fits-every dietary proposal and perceives the significance of fitting sustenance to individual necessities.

Home grown medication and herbal treatments are likewise embraced in comprehensive consideration, drawing on the recuperating properties of plants to help wellbeing and prosperity. Many societies have a rich history of involving spices for restorative purposes, and comprehensive consideration incorporates this customary information with present day proof based rehearses.

Natural cures might be utilized to address explicit side effects, support invulnerable capability, or improve generally speaking imperativeness. Notwithstanding, it is fundamental for medical services suppliers to have a thorough comprehension of home grown medication to guarantee protected and compelling reconciliation into patient consideration.

Besides, the brain body association is a focal principle of comprehensive consideration, perceiving that psychological and close to home prosperity significantly impacts actual wellbeing. Incorporating mental and daily reassurance into medical care includes tending to pressure, uneasiness, wretchedness, and other emotional well-being concerns. Psychosocial mediations, directing, and support bunches assume a critical part in advancing mental prosperity and improving the general personal satisfaction for people confronting wellbeing challenges.

Strong treatments incorporate a large number of mediations intended to mitigate side effects, upgrade prosperity, and work on the general personal satisfaction for patients. These treatments are much of the time utilized close by traditional clinical medicines to address the physical, profound, and social parts of wellbeing. They are especially significant in persistent and difficult sicknesses, where overseeing side effects and upgrading personal satisfaction are foremost.

Palliative consideration is a foundation of steady treatments, zeroing in on giving help from the side effects and stress of a difficult disease. It isn't restricted to end-of-life care however can be incorporated into the general consideration plan from the hour of analysis. Palliative consideration expects to work on the patient's solace, improve correspondence with medical services suppliers, and include the patient in choices about their consideration. This approach lines up with all encompassing consideration standards, perceiving the significance of tending to the complex necessities of people confronting difficult diseases.

Active recuperations, including physiotherapy and word related treatment, are fundamental parts of steady consideration. These treatments center around enhancing actual capability, overseeing side effects like torment and weakness, and working on by and large portability and autonomy. Coordinating active recuperations into the consideration plan is especially significant in conditions that influence actual working, like malignant growth, ongoing torment, and neurological problems.

Integral and elective treatments, like needle therapy, rub treatment, and chiropractic care, are progressively perceived as important increments to strong consideration. These treatments address different side effects, including agony, queasiness, and nervousness, and are much of the time generally welcomed by patients looking for a more comprehensive and patient-focused way to deal with their consideration. While the proof for a few reciprocal treatments is as yet developing, numerous people report critical advantages, underlining the significance of giving a different scope of strong choices.

Music treatment, workmanship treatment, and other expressive treatments add to the close to home and mental parts of steady consideration. These imaginative intercessions offer people confronting wellbeing challenges a method for self-articulation, close to home delivery, and adapting. Taking part in creative exercises can advance a feeling of strengthening, decrease pressure, and improve in general prosperity. Strong consideration perceives the helpful worth of imaginative articulation in advancing mental and close to home wellbeing.

In the domain of malignant growth care, the joining of comprehensive methodologies and steady treatments is especially pertinent. Malignant growth, a diverse and frequently life changing conclusion, requires an extensive model that tends to the physical and profound cost of the sickness and its therapy. All encompassing consideration in oncology includes fitting treatment plans to the singular's requirements, taking into account the effect on generally speaking prosperity, and perceiving the significance of survivorship and personal satisfaction.

Strong treatments assume a basic part in dealing with the results of malignant growth treatment. For instance, people going through chemotherapy might encounter sickness, weakness, and torment. Incorporating steady treatments like needle therapy, rub, and nourishing help can mitigate these side effects, upgrade therapy resilience, and work on the general personal satisfaction during disease treatment.

Additionally, comprehensive consideration in malignant growth therapy stretches out to survivorship and tending to the drawn out impacts of disease and its treatment. Survivorship care plans consider the physical, profound, and social parts of life after disease, underscoring continuous wellbeing, follow-up care, and backing for people changing back to their day to day routines. Incorporating strong treatments into survivorship care adds to a comprehensive and patient-focused approach that perceives the extraordinary necessities and objectives of malignant growth survivors.

The job of the medical care group is crucial in coordinating all encompassing consideration and strong treatments into traditional clinical methodologies. A cooperative and multidisciplinary approach includes medical care suppliers, including doctors, attendants, specialists, and guides, cooperating to address the different necessities of people confronting wellbeing challenges. Correspondence and coordination among colleagues are fundamental to guarantee a consistent and incorporated care insight for the patient.

Moreover, instruction and preparing are essential parts of effective reconciliation. Medical services suppliers need a strong comprehension of all encompassing standards, steady treatments, and proof based practices to integrate these methodologies into patient consideration really. Continuous schooling guarantees that medical care experts stay informed about arising research, progresses in integrative medication, and the advancing scene of strong consideration.

Patient training and strengthening are similarly significant in the mix of comprehensive consideration and strong treatments. Illuminating patients about the accessible choices, expected advantages, and dangers permits them to settle on informed conclusions about their consideration. Empowering open correspondence and joint effort between medical services suppliers and patients encourages a feeling of organization, advancing shared navigation and patient-focused care.

8.3 Highlighting successful patient-centered approaches

Fruitful patient-focused approaches in medical care exhibit a takeoff from customary models that focus on a sickness driven concentration to models that focus on the remarkable requirements, values, and inclinations of individual patients. These methodologies stress coordinated effort, open correspondence, and shared navigation, encouraging a more comprehensive and customized medical care climate. A few instances of fruitful patient-focused approaches across different medical services settings feature the positive effect of putting the patient at the focal point of care.

One outstanding model is the execution of patient-focused clinical homes (PCMHs). PCMHs are essential consideration rehearses that rearrange and upgrade the conveyance of care to stress the patient-supplier relationship and spotlight on extensive, facilitated, and open consideration. These models frequently include care groups, including doctors, medical attendants, and other medical care experts, working cooperatively to address the different necessities of patients.

In a patient-focused clinical home, patients have an assigned essential consideration supplier who fills in as the main issue of contact for their medical care needs. This supplier arranges all parts of the patient's consideration, including preventive administrations, constant infection the executives, and references to subject matter experts. The accentuation on progression of care and a group based approach adds to a more thorough comprehension of the patient's wellbeing and works with additional customized and proactive intercessions.

Besides, PCMHs frequently influence innovation to upgrade correspondence and patient commitment. Electronic wellbeing records (EHRs) empower consistent data dividing between care colleagues and enable patients to get to their wellbeing data, speak with their suppliers, and effectively partake in direction. The utilization of secure informing, telehealth administrations, and patient entries upholds continuous correspondence and advances a patient-focused way to deal with medical services conveyance.

Another fruitful patient-focused approach includes shared dynamic in disease care. Disease treatment choices frequently include complex contemplations, including possible advantages, gambles, and the effect on the patient's personal satisfaction. Shared direction recognizes that patients bring significant bits of knowledge into their own inclinations, values, and objectives, coming to them dynamic members in conclusions about their consideration.

Choice guides, instructive materials, and worked with conversations among patients and medical care suppliers are key parts of shared direction. These instruments assist patients with grasping their analysis, treatment choices, and expected results, permitting them to pursue choices that line up with their qualities and inclinations. Fruitful execution of shared dynamic in malignant growth care requires medical services suppliers to establish a climate that energizes open correspondence, regards patient independence, and encourages a cooperative dynamic cycle.

Besides, effective patient-focused approaches are apparent in the mix of patient-detailed results (Aces) into routine clinical consideration. Geniuses catch data straightforwardly from patients about their side effects, useful status, and personal satisfaction. By integrating Geniuses into clinical evaluations, medical services suppliers gain significant bits of knowledge into the patient's insight, considering a more all encompassing comprehension of their wellbeing and prosperity.

The precise assortment of Geniuses gives a stage to progressing correspondence among patients and medical services suppliers. It empowers early discovery of side effects or difficulties, taking into account convenient mediations and changes in accordance with the consideration plan. Effective execution of Masters requires the joining of normalized estimation apparatuses, work processes for gathering and investigating Star information, and components for integrating patient-revealed data into clinical independent direction.

In psychological well-being care, cooperative consideration models embody fruitful patient-focused approaches. Cooperative consideration includes a group based approach that coordinates emotional wellness experts into essential consideration settings. This model perceives areas of strength for the among mental and actual wellbeing and expects to address the two perspectives inside a solitary, facilitated care structure.

In cooperative consideration, a group comprising of essential consideration suppliers, conduct wellbeing trained professionals, and care chiefs cooperate to survey and deal with the patient's psychological well-being necessities. This approach guarantees that emotional well-being is coordinated into routine essential consideration, decreasing the shame related with looking for emotional wellness benefits and further developing admittance to convenient and extensive consideration.

Furthermore, patient commitment methodologies, for example, shared independent direction and self-administration support, are basic parts of fruitful cooperative consideration models. These systems engage patients to effectively partake in choices about their emotional wellness treatment, put forth customized objectives, and foster abilities to really deal with their circumstances. By consolidating patients as accomplices in their consideration, cooperative consideration models add to further developed results and patient fulfillment in emotional wellness settings.

In the domain of persistent illness the executives, effective patient-focused approaches are exemplified by drives that influence innovation to improve self-administration and advance patient commitment. Portable wellbeing (mHealth) applications, wearable gadgets, and remote checking apparatuses engage patients to screen their wellbeing, track side effects, and speak with their medical care suppliers continuously.

For example, patients with diabetes can utilize portable applications to log blood glucose levels, track dietary decisions, and get customized input on their self-administration endeavors. Likewise, people with hypertension can profit from remote checking gadgets that permit medical care suppliers to follow pulse drifts and change therapy designs as needs be. These advancements empower patients to partake in their consideration, prompting worked on self-adequacy and better administration of constant circumstances effectively.

Effective patient-focused approaches are additionally clear in drives that address wellbeing abberations and advance social skill in medical services conveyance. Perceiving the different necessities of patient populaces, especially those from underestimated networks, requires a promise to disposing of differences in access, nature of care, and wellbeing results.

Socially capable consideration includes understanding and regarding the social convictions, values, and inclinations of patients. This incorporates contemplations like language, wellbeing proficiency, and social customs. Medical care associations that focus on social skill carry out preparing programs for staff, give language benefits, and draw in with local area associations to guarantee that care is comprehensive and receptive to the assorted necessities of the populace they serve.

Besides, effective patient-focused approaches stretch out past individual experiences with medical care suppliers to incorporate the general medical care framework. Patient and family warning committees, where patients and their families effectively take part in molding strategies, systems, and quality improvement drives, represent a guarantee to patient-focused care at the hierarchical level.

These warning gatherings give a stage to patients to share their encounters, viewpoints, and suggestions with medical care initiative. This joint effort guarantees that the patient's voice is heard in dynamic cycles, adding to the ceaseless improvement of medical care administrations. Effective patient-focused associations effectively look for and esteem patient information, remembering it as fundamental for giving superior grade, patient-focused care.

All in all, fruitful patient-focused approaches in medical care are portrayed by a shift from illness driven models to those that focus on the extraordinary necessities, values, and inclinations of individual patients. Models, for example, patient-focused clinical homes, shared dynamic in malignant growth care, mix of patient-announced results, cooperative consideration models in

emotional well-being, innovation empowered ongoing sickness the executives, and drives advancing social ability feature the different manners by which patient-focused care is being carried out across different medical services settings. These methodologies focus on joint effort, open correspondence, and shared independent direction, at last prompting more comprehensive, customized, and successful medical care conveyance.

Patient-focused approaches in medical services have become progressively perceived as urgent procedures for conveying excellent and sympathetic clinical consideration. This change in outlook implies a takeoff from conventional models that frequently focus on illness driven points of view and supplier driven direction. All things considered, patient-focused approaches stress the significance of fitting medical services to the one of a kind requirements, values, and inclinations of individual patients, cultivating a cooperative and comprehensive medical care climate.

At the center of patient-focused care is the affirmation that patients are specialists in their own lives. This acknowledgment advances dynamic patient commitment to their consideration, accentuating shared navigation and the customization of treatment intends to line up with the patient's objectives and inclinations. Patient-focused care, on a very basic level, puts the patient at the focal point of the medical services insight, upholding for an all encompassing comprehension of wellbeing that rises above the simple shortfall of sickness.

Powerful correspondence fills in as a key part in quiet focused approaches. Open and straightforward correspondence fabricates trust, upgrades understanding, and enables patients to partake in choices about their wellbeing effectively. Undivided attention, recognizing patient worries, and answering sympathetically to their requirements are necessary parts of powerful correspondence in persistent focused care.

Shared direction addresses a basic component of patient-focused care. This cooperative cycle includes medical services suppliers and patients cooperating to settle on conclusions about the patient's consideration. Shared direction perceives that patients bring important bits of knowledge into their own inclinations, values, and ways of life, which can fundamentally affect the outcome of treatment plans. Through shared navigation, patients become dynamic accomplices in their medical services venture, adding to a more customized and viable consideration experience.

Moreover, patient-focused care stretches out past individual connections to incorporate the general medical services framework. It includes a pledge to social capability, perceiving and regarding the variety of patients concerning their experiences, convictions, and values. Medical services associations that embrace patient-focused approaches effectively try to dispense with wellbeing variations and elevate value in admittance to mind.

Executing patient-focused care requires a foundational shift in the way of life of medical services conveyance. This change includes changes in strategies, methods, and the general attitude of medical care suppliers and associations. Embracing patient-focused approaches frequently requires a takeoff from the customary paternalistic model of medical care towards a model that values cooperation, regard, and inclusivity.

In pragmatic terms, patient-focused care includes fitting clinical medicines to the special requirements and inclinations of individual patients. This might incorporate thinking about a patient's social foundation, financial status, and individual convictions while fostering a consideration plan. In doing as such, medical care suppliers can make more powerful and patient-accommodating mediations that reverberate with the singular's way of life and values.

The idea of patient-focused care additionally perceives the significance of tending to the actual parts of wellbeing as well as the profound, social, and mental aspects. This all encompassing methodology thinks about the effect of sickness on a patient's general prosperity and personal satisfaction. Subsequently, patient-focused care might include incorporating psychosocial support, emotional well-being administrations, and assets for patients and their families.

Patient-focused care is especially applicable in ongoing illness the executives, where long haul commitment and coordinated effort among patients and medical services suppliers are urgent. Constant circumstances frequently require continuous self-administration, and patients assume a focal part in settling on conclusions about their consideration on an everyday premise. In such cases, patient-focused approaches enable people to become dynamic members in their wellbeing the board, encouraging a feeling of independence and control.

The advantages of patient-focused care stretch out past the singular patient to the medical services framework in general. Studies have shown that patient-focused approaches add to worked on understanding fulfillment, adherence to treatment plans, and wellbeing results. By including patients in their consideration, medical care suppliers can likewise improve proficiency and lessen medical care costs by keeping away from superfluous mediations and hospitalizations.

Notwithstanding the various benefits of patient-focused care, its far and wide reception faces difficulties inside the ongoing medical services scene. One huge snag is the settled in custom of the various leveled supplier patient relationship, where the medical care proficient is many times seen as the sole power. Moving towards a more cooperative model requires a social change that difficulties existing power elements and advances a common perspective of skill.

Another test includes time imperatives inside medical services settings. The conventional model of care frequently focuses on proficiency, with restricted time for patient associations. Executing patient-focused care requires apportioning adequate time for significant discussions, undivided attention, and shared direction. This requires a reconsideration of medical services conveyance models and asset portion to help these fundamental parts of patient-focused care.

The incorporation of innovation into medical services presents the two open doors and difficulties for patient-focused approaches. On one hand, innovation can upgrade correspondence, work with remote observing, and give patients important wellbeing data. Then again, the rising dependence on electronic wellbeing records and mechanized frameworks may unintentionally depersonalize the patient-supplier relationship. Finding some kind of harmony among innovation and human-focused care is critical for the effective execution of patient-focused approaches.

Schooling and preparing are significant in encouraging a medical services labor force that embraces patient-focused care. Medical care experts need to foster abilities in viable correspondence, social capability, and shared navigation. Moreover, ingraining a patient-focused mentality requires progressing instruction to stay up with developing medical care rehearses and the mix of new proof based approaches.

The patient's viewpoint on their medical services experience is a key measurement in assessing the outcome of patient-focused care. Patient-announced results (Experts) give important bits of knowledge into the effect of sickness and therapy on the patient's personal satisfaction. These results can illuminate medical care suppliers about the adequacy regarding intercessions and guide changes in accordance with therapy plans in view of the patient's insight.

Patient-focused approaches are especially significant with regards to preventive consideration and wellbeing advancement. Engaging people to play a functioning job in keeping up with their wellbeing can add to the counteraction of sicknesses and the advancement of generally prosperity. This proactive methodology includes teaching patients about solid way of life decisions, preventive screenings, and early discovery of potential medical problems.

The idea of patient-focused care lines up with the standards of individual focused medication, which stresses the significance of figuring out patients as interesting people with their own accounts, values, and objectives. Individual focused medication rises above the reductionist methodology that sees patients exclusively from the perspective of their infections. All things considered, it perceives the interconnectedness of physical, mental, and social variables in forming a singular's wellbeing.

Firmly connected with individual focused medication is the idea of account medication, which highlights the meaning of narrating in medical services. Perceiving that disease isn't simply an organic peculiarity yet in addition a story experience, account medication urges medical services suppliers to stand by listening to patients' accounts, figure out their points of view, and coordinate these accounts into the more extensive setting of care.

The reception of patient-focused care isn't restricted to explicit clinical fortes yet is pertinent across many disciplines. Whether in essential consideration, specialty facilities, or medical clinic settings, patient-focused approaches improve the general nature of care and add to positive patient encounters. This inclusivity builds up the possibility that patient-focused care is an essential part of medical services conveyance instead of a specific practice.

Patient commitment is a focal precept of patient-focused care, underscoring the dynamic contribution of people in their medical services venture. Drawn in patients are bound to stick to treatment plans, partake in shared navigation, and take responsibility for wellbeing. Medical care suppliers can work with patient commitment by cultivating a cooperative and enabling climate that esteems the info and viewpoints of people.

The idea of patient-focused care stretches out past the clinical setting to envelop the more extensive medical services biological system, including wellbeing strategy and promotion. Promotion for patient-focused approaches includes perceiving patients as partners in medical care navigation and guaranteeing their portrayal in conversations about medical care conveyance, exploration, and asset designation. Strategies that focus on quiet focused approaches add to a more responsive and evenhanded medical care framework.

Chapter 9

Future Prospects and Challenges

What's to come is a complex embroidery woven with the strings of mechanical advancement, cultural development, and ecological difficulties. As we stand on the incline representing things to come, looking into the huge obscure, urgent to evaluate the imminent directions lie ahead and the difficulties that might go with them.

Perhaps of the most significant and groundbreaking power forming what's in store is innovation. The quick progression of man-made consciousness (simulated intelligence), AI, and computerization proclaims another period where the limits between the advanced and actual universes obscure. The joining of brilliant innovations into different aspects of our lives, from savvy homes to shrewd urban communities, guarantees uncommon accommodation and effectiveness.

In the domain of medical care, the assembly of innovation and science opens up roads for customized medication, hereditary treatments, and imaginative analytic apparatuses. Accuracy medication, customized to a person's hereditary cosmetics, can possibly alter treatment draws near, furnishing designated arrangements with negligible incidental effects. Additionally, the appearance of telemedicine and wearable wellbeing gadgets works with far off understanding observing, improving openness to medical care administrations.

The ascent of sustainable power sources remains as an encouraging sign despite environmental change and ecological debasement. Sunlight based, wind, and other supportable energy innovations offer the commitment of a cleaner and greener future. As countries overall progressively focus on environmentally friendly power drives, the change to a low-carbon economy picks up speed, giving a brief look at a more reasonable tomorrow.

Be that as it may, close by these promising possibilities, a sorry excuse for difficulties poses a potential threat. The moral ramifications of artificial intelligence and robotization, for example, bring up issues about work removal, protection attack, and the grouping of force. The financial texture might go through huge changes as specific positions become old, requiring the reconsideration of schooling and labor force preparing projects to furnish people with abilities pertinent to the advanced age.

Additionally, the clouded side of mechanical advancement appears as online protection dangers. As our reliance on interconnected frameworks develops, so does the weakness to cyberattacks. Shielding touchy information, basic framework, and individual security turns into a continuous fight, requiring steady advancement in network protection measures.

With regards to globalization, what's in store holds both the commitment of improved worldwide participation and the test of exploring international intricacies. The interconnectedness of economies, societies, and social orders cultivates open doors for joint effort in resolving worldwide issues, for example, environmental change, pandemics, and destitution. On the other side, international strains and epic showdowns present dangers to soundness, possibly obstructing progress on shared difficulties.

Environmental change stays an impressive test that requests dire consideration and purposeful endeavors. Increasing temperatures, outrageous climate occasions, and natural disturbances highlight the requirement for maintainable practices and relief techniques. The change to a carbon-impartial world requires composed activity on a worldwide scale, with countries, ventures, and people focusing on lessening fossil fuel byproducts and embracing eco-accommodating practices.

In the domain of room investigation, what's to come entices with the commitment of new revelations and extended human presence past Earth. As privately owned businesses and worldwide space organizations put resources into aggressive missions to Mars, the Moon, and then some, the possibility of interplanetary colonization turns into an unmistakable objective. Nonetheless, the difficulties of long-term space travel, life emotionally supportive networks, and the moral contemplations of extraterrestrial investigation go with these advanced undertakings.

The segment scene is going through huge movements, with maturing populaces in certain districts and a young lump in others. The ramifications of these segment changes stretch out to medical care, social administrations, and financial elements.

Maturing social orders wrestle with medical care requests and benefits frameworks, while young populaces face the difficulties of schooling, business, and guaranteeing a practical future for a long time into the future.

Training itself remains at a junction despite mechanical headways. The conventional model of instruction is being reshaped by internet learning, virtual homerooms, and computerized accreditations. The democratization of training through web-based stages offers admittance to information on a worldwide scale, yet issues of computerized partition and the nature of online instruction present difficulties to evenhanded learning open doors.

The nexus of bioethics and biotechnology brings up significant issues about the constraints of logical mediation in the normal request. CRISPR quality altering innovation, for example, makes the way for uncommon conceivable outcomes in adjusting the human genome. While this holds potential for annihilating hereditary infections, it additionally raises moral issues in regards to architect children, hereditary improvements, and the unexpected outcomes of altering the structure blocks of life.

In the monetary scene, the ascent of decentralized finance (DeFi) and blockchain innovation challenges customary monetary frameworks. Digital currencies, brilliant agreements, and decentralized applications offer options in contrast to concentrated banking and administration structures. In any case, administrative vulnerabilities, security concerns, and the potential for monetary unsteadiness go with the problematic power of blockchain development.

The fate of work is going through a change in perspective, driven via robotization, distant innovations, and the gig economy. The customary all day office model is giving way to adaptable work game plans, far off coordinated effort, and a gig-based labor force. While this cultivates spryness and balance between fun and serious activities, it likewise brings up issues about employer stability, social security nets, and the prosperity of people in a quickly developing workplace.

Medical services frameworks overall face the test of adjusting to the advancing scene of infections, including the continuous fight against pandemics. The Coronavirus pandemic, a worldwide emergency that rose above borders, featured the weaknesses in general wellbeing framework and the requirement for readiness and global participation. What's in store calls for strong medical care frameworks equipped for answering arising dangers and guaranteeing impartial admittance to clinical assets.

The social and cultural texture is being rewoven by the powers of globalization, movement, and mechanical interconnectedness. Social trade and variety carry wealth to social orders, yet they additionally flash discussions about character, digestion, and the conservation of social legacy.

Exploring the sensitive harmony between social transparency and the safeguarding of individual and aggregate personalities represents a consistent test for social orders all over the planet.

As we look into the future, the job of administration and political frameworks turns out to be progressively basic. The difficulties of guaranteeing straightforwardness, responsibility, and powerful authority are complemented in a world confronting mind boggling and interconnected issues. Finding some kind of harmony between individual opportunities and aggregate prosperity stays a continuous undertaking for policymakers and residents the same.

The speeding up speed of progress in the mechanical scene requests a reconsideration of moral systems and lawful structures. Inquiries concerning information protection, algorithmic inclination, and the dependable turn of events and utilization of arising advancements require nuanced and versatile methodologies. The advancement of moral rules and worldwide norms becomes basic to dependably explore the strange regions of the computerized age.

Natural manageability arises as a foundation for the future, with the need to address environmental change, biodiversity misfortune, and asset consumption. The change to round economies, sustainable power sources, and eco-accommodating practices becomes a natural need as well as a monetary objective. Offsetting financial development with biological conservation requires creative arrangements and a pledge to maintainable turn of events.

In the domain of man-made brainpower, the moral contemplations of making independent frameworks that can pursue choices autonomously raise complex moral issues. As simulated intelligence applications become more coordinated into basic regions like medical services, money, and policing, decency, straightforwardness, and responsibility in algorithmic navigation becomes principal. Finding some kind of harmony among development and moral shields is really difficult for the eventual fate of simulated intelligence.

The crossing point of innovation and human expansion opens up opportunities for improving human abilities. From mind machine points of interaction to wearable innovations, the beneficial interaction among people and machines holds potential for clinical leap forwards, mental upgrades, and new types of correspondence. Notwithstanding, moral worries with respect to protection, assent, and the ramifications of obscuring the lines among human and machine wait not too far off.

In the international field, the ascent of new worldwide powers and the moving elements of global relations present the two amazing open doors and dangers. The development of multipolar world request difficulties customary ideas of worldwide administration and discretion. Finding some kind of harmony between public interests and worldwide participation turns into a fragile dance, with issues like exchange strains, regional debates, and the journey for vital predominance molding the international scene.

The phantom of worldwide wellbeing emergencies, exemplified by the Coronavirus pandemic, highlights the requirement for an organized and proactive way to deal with general wellbeing. What's in store requires vigorous worldwide wellbeing framework, early admonition frameworks, and cooperative examination endeavors to address arising irresistible sicknesses. The examples gained from the pandemic stress the interconnectedness of the world and the significance of fortitude in confronting normal difficulties.

In the domain of energy, the change to sustainable sources and the mission for energy proficiency become the overwhelming focus. The improvement of cutting edge energy capacity advances, lattice modernization, and practical transportation arrangements becomes urgent in accomplishing a carbon-nonpartisan future. Nonetheless, the difficulties of energy stockpiling, discontinuity of sustainable sources, and the current framework's latency present obstacles in the race towards a practical energy worldview.

The eventual fate of transportation is on the cusp of an upheaval, with electric vehicles, independent driving innovation, and creative metropolitan versatility arrangements reshaping the manner in which we move. The commitment of cleaner and more productive transportation frameworks comes connected at the hip with challenges connected with foundation improvement, administrative systems, and cultural acknowledgment of groundbreaking advancements.

In the rural area, what's to come holds the commitment of accuracy cultivating, feasible practices, and creative answers for address food security challenges. The reconciliation of innovation, like robots, sensors, and information investigation, improves horticultural effectiveness and asset use. Notwithstanding, the need to offset innovative headways with moral contemplations, ecological stewardship, and social value stays a basic part representing things to come of food creation.

The combination of nanotechnology, biotechnology, and data innovation opens up new outskirts in logical disclosure and advancement. From designated drug conveyance frameworks to cutting edge materials with remarkable properties, the potential applications are immense. In any case, moral worries with respect to the dependable utilization of these advances, expected gambles, and long haul ecological effects require cautious thought and moral oversight.

In the social domain, what's to come allures with the commitment of inclusivity, correspondence, and civil rights. Developments pushing for orientation correspondence, racial equity, and LGBTQ+ freedoms pick up speed, testing cultural standards and cultivating a more comprehensive world. Nonetheless, well established fundamental imbalances, social obstruction, and the requirement for foundational change present impressive difficulties on the way towards an all the more and evenhanded society.

Instruction, as a foundation of cultural advancement, faces the test of adjusting to the developing requirements representing things to come. The customary schooling model, intended for a modern time society, wrestles with the requests of a quickly changing computerized scene. What's to come requires a reconsidering of instruction, integrating decisive reasoning, inventiveness, and versatility to plan people for the difficulties and chances of the 21st hundred years.

In the journey for economical turn of events, the idea of a round economy acquires conspicuousness. Moving from a straight model of creation and utilization to a roundabout one, where assets are reused, reused, and recovered, becomes basic for relieving natural effect. Be that as it may, the progress to a round economy requires fundamental changes, coordinated effort across enterprises, and a change in customer conduct.

The eventual fate of global participation faces the double difficulties of rising patriotism and the basic for aggregate activity. Worldwide issues, for example, environmental change, pandemics, and financial imbalance request cooperative endeavors on a scale never seen. Finding some kind of harmony between public interests and worldwide obligations turns into a characterizing component representing things to come international scene.

The domains of computer generated reality (VR) and increased reality (AR) hold the commitment of vivid encounters, changing diversion, training, and different enterprises. From virtual homerooms to expanded working environment conditions, the joining of these innovations reshapes the manner in which we connect with the computerized world. Notwithstanding, moral worries in regards to security, the obscuring of the real world and virtuality, and the potential for fixation go with the groundbreaking force of VR and AR.

The eventual fate of a majority rules government faces difficulties in exploring the intricacies of a computerized age. The ascent of deception, algorithmic control, and the effect of virtual entertainment on open talk highlight the requirement for a reconsideration of majority rule processes. Shielding the honesty of decisions, guaranteeing straightforwardness in administration, and encouraging an educated populace become pivotal parts of forming the fate of vote based social orders.

The mission for counterfeit general insight (AGI), a type of man-made intelligence that can comprehend, learn, and apply information across different spaces, presents both unimaginable open doors and existential dangers. The advancement of AGI could alter enterprises, take care of mind boggling issues, and raise human capacities. Nonetheless, the moral contemplations, possible abuse, and the requirement for vigorous protections against unseen side-effects request cautious and capable turn of events.

The eventual fate of room investigation holds the commitment of wandering past our divine area, with aggressive missions to far off planets and the investigation of exoplanets that might hold onto indications of extraterrestrial life. The mission to disentangle the secrets of the universe grows how we might interpret the universe and our place in it. In any case, the difficulties of room travel, the moral contemplations of divine colonization, and the capable utilization of room assets require cautious consultation.

9.1 Exploration of emerging trends in cancer research and treatment

The scene of disease exploration and therapy is developing quickly, set apart by forward leaps in grasping the sub-atomic underpinnings of malignant growth, creative helpful methodologies, and a developing accentuation on customized medication. As we dive into the investigation of arising patterns in disease exploration and treatment, it becomes apparent that what's to come holds guarantee for additional successful and designated mediations, while likewise introducing difficulties that request clever fixes.

Progressions in genomics have been a main impetus in unwinding the intricacies of disease. The coming of cutting edge sequencing advances has empowered analysts to dissect the whole genomic scene of malignant growth cells, distinguishing key transformations, modifications, and flagging pathways that drive tumorigenesis. This more profound comprehension of the hereditary premise of malignant growth has prepared for accuracy medication, fitting treatment methodologies in view of the novel hereditary profile of every patient's cancer.

Immunotherapy stands apart as a groundbreaking methodology in malignant growth treatment. Outfitting the force of the resistant framework to perceive and kill disease cells, immunotherapy has shown amazing outcome in different tumors. Designated spot inhibitors, Vehicle White blood cell treatment, and malignant growth immunizations are among the immunotherapeutic techniques that have shown viability in certain patients, prompting strong reactions and, now and again, long haul reduction. The continuous investigation of novel immunotherapeutic targets and blend treatments holds extraordinary commitment for growing the relevance of immunotherapy across various malignant growth types.

The field of fluid biopsy has arisen as a painless strategy for recognizing and checking disease. Examining circling cancer DNA (ctDNA) or other biomarkers in blood tests gives a constant preview of the growth's hereditary cosmetics, considering early location, checking therapy reaction, and identifying negligible leftover illness. Fluid biopsy can possibly reform malignant growth diagnostics, offering a less obtrusive option in contrast to conventional tissue biopsies and empowering more successive and dynamic checking of the illness.

Man-made consciousness (artificial intelligence) and AI have become essential devices in disease examination and treatment. The capacity of artificial intelligence calculations to investigate immense datasets, including genomic data, clinical imaging, and clinical records, works with more exact analysis, visualization, and treatment arranging.

Artificial intelligence driven approaches are supporting the ID of novel medication targets, foreseeing patient reactions to treatments, and improving treatment methodologies, introducing a time of information driven accuracy oncology.

The investigation of the growth microenvironment has acquired noticeable quality in grasping disease movement and treatment opposition. The mind boggling interaction between malignant growth cells, resistant cells, stromal cells, and the extracellular framework impacts cancer conduct. Focusing on parts of the cancer microenvironment, like resistant designated spot particles and angiogenic pathways, offers new roads for restorative intercession. Procedures pointed toward adjusting the insusceptible reaction inside the cancer microenvironment intend to defeat immuno-suppression and upgrade the viability of immunotherapy.

Fluid biopsy, a harmless strategy for distinguishing disease, is getting momentum in the journey for early determination and observing of treatment reactions. Breaking down coursing cancer DNA (ctDNA) shed by growths into the circulatory system gives a dynamic and ongoing perspective on the genomic modifications present in the cancer. This approach holds incredible commitment for distinguishing diseases at prior stages, checking treatment reactions, and recognizing the development of obstruction changes. As fluid biopsy innovations keep on propelling, they might become basic parts of routine disease care, offering a less intrusive option in contrast to conventional tissue biopsies.

The incorporation of multi-omics information, consolidating data from genomics, transcriptomics, proteomics, and metabolomics, empowers an exhaustive comprehension of the sub-atomic scene of malignant growth. This comprehensive methodology gives experiences into the many-sided transaction of hereditary, epigenetic, and ecological variables adding to disease improvement. By interpreting the complex atomic organizations overseeing tumorigenesis, scientists can recognize new restorative targets and biomarkers, preparing for more exact and powerful malignant growth medicines.

In the domain of designated treatments, the investigation of engineered lethality has arisen as a promising technique. Engineered lethality takes advantage of the idea that the concurrent interruption of two explicit qualities or pathways is deadly to malignant growth cells yet not to typical cells. This approach takes into consideration the particular focusing of disease cells holding onto explicit hereditary changes while saving sound tissues. The distinguishing proof of engineered deadly communications offers another worldview for creating designated treatments with expanded particularity and decreased askew impacts.

The microbiome, containing trillions of microorganisms living in the human body, has been ensnared in affecting malignant growth advancement and treatment results. The stomach microbiome, specifically, assumes a urgent part in tweaking the resistant framework and medication digestion.

Understanding the many-sided connection between the microbiome and disease holds potential for enhancing immunotherapy reactions, moderating therapy related poison levels, and in any event, affecting malignant growth vulnerability. Continuous exploration looks to disentangle the intricacies of the microbiome-malignant growth hub and saddle its remedial potential.

Chasing more compelling malignant growth therapies, analysts are investigating the one of a kind weaknesses of disease cells. Metabolic weaknesses, specifically, stand out, as malignant growth cells frequently display particular metabolic profiles contrasted with ordinary cells. Focusing on unambiguous metabolic pathways basic for disease cell endurance and expansion offers a clever remedial methodology. Systems pointed toward upsetting supplement take-up, changing energy digestion, or taking advantage of metabolic conditions give another wilderness in the advancement of hostile to disease treatments.

The idea of fluid biopsy, which includes dissecting flowing growth DNA (ctDNA) or other biomarkers in blood tests, is upsetting disease diagnostics and observing. Dissimilar to customary tissue biopsies, fluid biopsy offers a painless and dynamic way to deal with evaluating the hereditary scene of growths. This strategy takes into consideration early malignant growth location, observing treatment reactions, and identifying insignificant leftover infection. As fluid biopsy innovations keep on propelling, they hold the possibility to change clinical practice by giving continuous experiences into the genomic development of growths.

Headways in disease immunotherapy have opened new roads for bridling the body's safe framework to target and wipe out malignant growth cells. Designated spot inhibitors, like PD-1 and PD-L1 inhibitors, have shown wonderful progress in specific diseases by delivering the brakes on resistant reactions. Vehicle Lymphocyte treatment, one more type of immunotherapy, includes designing a patient's own White blood cells to perceive and go after malignant growth cells. The continuous investigation of novel insusceptible designated spots, mix immunotherapies, and defeating opposition systems means to expand the materialness of immunotherapy across a more extensive range of malignant growths.

The union of immunotherapy and accuracy medication has prompted the advancement of customized disease antibodies. These immunizations are intended to invigorate the patient's insusceptible framework to perceive and target explicit growth antigens, customized to the singular's novel disease profile. Customized malignant growth antibodies hold the possibility to improve the resistant reaction against cancers while limiting askew impacts. This approach addresses a change in outlook towards individualized disease therapy methodologies, where the resistant framework turns into a designated weapon against the particular sub-atomic elements of every patient's malignant growth.

The combination of man-made consciousness (simulated intelligence) and AI into malignant growth examination and treatment can possibly reform how we approach the illness. Computer based intelligence calculations can examine enormous datasets, including genomic data,

clinical imaging, and clinical records, to recognize examples and connections that might escape human investigation. In diagnostics, simulated intelligence driven apparatuses can help with deciphering complex genomic information, working on the exactness of malignant growth subtype order and forecast expectation. Furthermore, in clinical imaging, artificial intelligence calculations help in the early discovery of cancers, empowering opportune mediation and further developed results.

The investigation of the growth microenvironment has given vital experiences into the powerful associations between disease cells and their encompassing milieu. The cancer microenvironment envelops insusceptible cells, fibroblasts, veins, and the extracellular network, all of which impact growth conduct and therapy reactions. Focusing on parts of the cancer microenvironment, like insusceptible designated spot particles and angiogenic pathways, has turned into a point of convergence for creating novel remedial procedures. By adjusting the invulnerable reaction inside the cancer microenvironment, analysts mean to improve the adequacy of immunotherapy and beaten opposition instruments.

The mission for manufactured lethality as a remedial technique includes recognizing blends of hereditary changes that are deadly to malignant growth cells. This approach considers the advancement of designated treatments that specifically exploit weaknesses in malignant growth cells while saving ordinary cells. Manufactured lethality has shown guarantee in different malignant growths, incorporating those with explicit hereditary transformations, for example, BRCA-changed cancers. The continuous investigation of engineered deadly associations holds potential for growing the collection of accuracy treatments, giving custom fitted therapies in light of the remarkable hereditary cosmetics of every patient's disease.

Multi-omics mix, which includes dissecting information from genomics, transcriptomics, proteomics, and metabolomics, gives a comprehensive comprehension of the sub-atomic scene of disease. This extensive methodology permits analysts to disentangle the unpredictable interaction of hereditary and natural variables adding to disease advancement. By interpreting the complex atomic organizations administering tumorigenesis, analysts can recognize new remedial targets and biomarkers, making ready for more exact and compelling malignant growth medicines. The reconciliation of multi-omics information addresses a change in perspective towards a frameworks science way to deal with malignant growth research.

The microbiome's part in disease advancement and treatment results is an arising area of examination. The stomach microbiome, specifically, has been embroiled in balancing the resistant framework and impacting reactions to disease immunotherapy. Understanding the mind boggling interaction between the microbiome and disease holds potential for enhancing therapy reactions, alleviating therapy related poison levels, and in any event, impacting malignant growth weakness. Progressing research looks to reveal the complicated connections between unambiguous microbial networks and different parts of disease science, making ready for microbiome-based mediations in malignant growth care.

Metabolic weaknesses in malignant growth cells have turned into a focal point of investigation for creating designated treatments. Disease cells frequently display particular metabolic profiles contrasted with typical cells, depending on unambiguous pathways for energy creation and biosynthesis. Focusing on these metabolic conditions offers a clever way to deal with upsetting disease cell endurance and expansion. Methodologies pointed toward restraining key metabolic chemicals, changing supplement accessibility, or taking advantage of metabolic weaknesses give another wilderness in the advancement of against disease treatments.

Chasing after more compelling malignant growth medicines, the idea of engineered lethality has acquired noticeable quality. Engineered lethality takes advantage of the possibility that the synchronous interruption of two explicit qualities or pathways is deadly to disease cells however not to typical cells. This approach considers the particular focusing of disease cells holding onto explicit hereditary modifications while saving sound tissues. The recognizable proof of manufactured deadly communications offers another worldview for creating designated treatments with expanded explicitness and diminished askew impacts.

The investigation of metabolic weaknesses in disease cells has prompted the advancement of designated treatments pointed toward upsetting explicit metabolic pathways fundamental for cancer development. Malignant growth cells frequently display changed digestion, depending on particular metabolic pathways to meet their energy and biosynthetic requirements. Focusing on these metabolic conditions offers an original way to deal with specifically repress malignant growth cell multiplication while saving ordinary cells. The continuous investigation of metabolic weaknesses holds guarantee for the improvement of imaginative treatments that exploit the interesting highlights of malignant growth cell digestion.

As malignant growth research keeps on propelling, the intermingling of immunotherapy and accuracy medication has prompted the improvement of customized disease antibodies. These antibodies are intended to invigorate the patient's invulnerable framework to perceive and target explicit growth antigens, custom-made to the singular's one of a kind disease profile. Customized disease immunizations address a change in outlook towards individualized malignant growth therapy techniques, where the resistant framework turns into a designated weapon against the particular sub-atomic highlights of every patient's disease.

The coordination of man-made reasoning (computer based intelligence) and AI into malignant growth exploration and treatment can possibly alter how we approach the sickness. Man-made intelligence calculations can examine huge datasets, including genomic data, clinical imaging, and clinical records, to distinguish examples and relationships that might escape human examination. In diagnostics, artificial intelligence driven apparatuses can help with deciphering complex genomic information, working on the precision of disease subtype characterization and guess expectation. Moreover, in clinical imaging, simulated intelligence calculations help in the early location of cancers, empowering ideal mediation and further developed results.

The investigation of the growth microenvironment has given significant experiences into the unique connections between disease cells and their encompassing milieu. The growth microenvironment envelops insusceptible cells, fibroblasts, veins, and the extracellular network, all of which impact cancer conduct and therapy reactions. Focusing on parts of the cancer microenvironment, like insusceptible designated spot particles and angiogenic pathways, has turned into a point of convergence for creating novel restorative methodologies. By adjusting the safe reaction inside the cancer microenvironment, specialists intend to upgrade the adequacy of immunotherapy and conquered obstruction instruments.

The microbiome's part in malignant growth advancement and treatment results is an arising area of examination. The stomach microbiome, specifically, has been embroiled in tweaking the resistant framework and impacting reactions to disease immunotherapy. Understanding the complicated interchange between the microbiome and malignant growth holds potential for improving therapy reactions, alleviating therapy related poison levels, and in any event, impacting disease helplessness. Continuous exploration tries to reveal the perplexing connections between unambiguous microbial networks and different parts of disease science, making ready for microbiome-based mediations in malignant growth care.

Metabolic weaknesses in disease cells have turned into a focal point of investigation for creating designated treatments. Disease cells frequently display particular metabolic profiles contrasted with typical cells, depending on unambiguous pathways for energy creation and biosynthesis. Focusing on these metabolic conditions offers a clever way to deal with upsetting malignant growth cell endurance and multiplication. Systems pointed toward restraining key metabolic chemicals, changing supplement accessibility, or taking advantage of metabolic weaknesses give another outskirts in the advancement of against malignant growth treatments.

Chasing after more compelling malignant growth medicines, the idea of engineered lethality has acquired noticeable quality. Engineered lethality takes advantage of the possibility that the synchronous interruption of two explicit qualities or pathways is deadly to disease cells however not to typical cells. This approach considers the particular focusing of disease cells holding onto explicit hereditary modifications while saving sound tissues. The recognizable proof of manufactured deadly communications offers another worldview for creating designated treatments with expanded explicitness and diminished askew impacts.

The investigation of metabolic weaknesses in disease cells has prompted the advancement of designated treatments pointed toward upsetting explicit metabolic pathways fundamental for cancer development. Malignant growth cells frequently display adjusted digestion, depending on unmistakable metabolic pathways to meet their energy and biosynthetic requirements. Focusing on these metabolic conditions offers an original way to deal with specifically repress malignant growth cell multiplication while saving typical cells.

The continuous investigation of metabolic weaknesses holds guarantee for the improvement of imaginative treatments that exploit the remarkable elements of malignant growth cell digestion.

As disease research keeps on propelling, the union of immunotherapy and accuracy medication has prompted the advancement of customized malignant growth antibodies. These antibodies are intended to invigorate the patient's safe framework to perceive and target explicit growth antigens, custom fitted to the singular's novel disease profile. Customized disease immunizations address a change in outlook towards individualized malignant growth therapy methodologies, where the safe framework turns into a designated weapon against the particular sub-atomic highlights of every patient's malignant growth.

The coordination of man-made brainpower (computer based intelligence) and AI into malignant growth exploration and treatment can possibly change how we approach the infection. Computer based intelligence calculations can examine enormous datasets, including genomic data, clinical imaging, and clinical records, to distinguish examples and connections that might evade human examination. In diagnostics, simulated intelligence driven devices can help with deciphering complex genomic information, working on the precision of malignant growth subtype characterization and visualization expectation. Furthermore, in clinical imaging, man-made intelligence calculations help in the early recognition of growths, empowering convenient mediation and further developed results.

9.2 Anticipated challenges and ethical considerations

As we explore the always developing scene of disease exploration and treatment, it is fundamental to perceive and expect the difficulties that go with these notable headways. Besides, moral contemplations assume a critical part in directing the dependable turn of events and utilization of arising advancements and restorative methodologies. Addressing these difficulties and moral worries is essential to guaranteeing that advancement in disease research isn't just logically sound yet additionally morally grounded.

One of the chief difficulties in the domain of disease exploration and therapy is the intrinsic intricacy and heterogeneity of malignant growth itself. Malignant growth is certainly not a solitary element; rather, it envelops a bunch of illnesses with different hereditary and sub-atomic qualities. While progressions in genomics and sub-atomic profiling have considered more exact grouping and designated treatments, the sheer variety of malignant growth types represents an impressive test. Fitting therapies to the particular hereditary modifications of every patient's growth requires a nuanced comprehension of the multifaceted sub-atomic scene, requiring continuous examination to disentangle the intricacies of various disease subtypes.

The approach of customized medication, driven by genomics and accuracy oncology, carries with it the test of openness and reasonableness. The expense of genomic profiling and designated treatments can be restrictively costly, restricting admittance to these state of the art

medicines for specific patient populaces. Guaranteeing evenhanded admittance to customized malignant growth care is a squeezing worry that requires mechanical progressions as well as strategy measures and global coordinated effort to overcome any barrier in medical services variations.

Immunotherapy, while proclaimed as a leap forward in malignant growth treatment, faces difficulties connected with solidness and obstruction. While certain patients experience amazing and strong reactions to immunotherapies, others might foster opposition after some time. Understanding the elements adding to treatment opposition and creating systems to beat these difficulties are basic for augmenting the drawn out viability of immunotherapy. Furthermore, overseeing resistant related unfavorable occasions, which can influence different organs, represents a clinical test that requires watchful observing and custom-made mediations.

In the domain of fluid biopsy, in spite of its commitment as a harmless demonstrative device, challenges exist concerning responsiveness, explicitness, and normalization.

Identifying follow measures of flowing growth DNA (ctDNA) in the circulation system requires exceptionally touchy procedures, and bogus up-sides or negatives can have critical clinical ramifications. Normalizing fluid biopsy methodology and laying out clear rules for translation and detailing are fundamental to guarantee the unwavering quality and precision of this arising symptomatic methodology.

The mix of man-made consciousness (artificial intelligence) and AI in disease research raises moral worries connected with information protection, predisposition, and interpretability. The utilization of immense datasets, including genomic data and patient records, presents dangers to individual security, and protecting delicate wellbeing information is of fundamental significance. In addition, the potential for predisposition in artificial intelligence calculations, particularly whenever prepared on datasets that are not agent of different populaces, raises worries about even-handed admittance to computer based intelligence driven advances. Guaranteeing straightforwardness and interpretability of artificial intelligence models is essential for incorporating trust and working with their capable joining into clinical practice.

In the investigation of the growth microenvironment, a test lies in unraveling the multifaceted exchange between various cell parts. The dynamic and complex nature of the growth microenvironment requires refined insightful ways to deal with grasp the crosstalk between disease cells, safe cells, and stromal parts. Besides, creating restorative mediations that specifically target parts of the cancer microenvironment without causing unseen side-effects or off-target impacts represents a huge logical and clinical test.

Moral contemplations in disease research stretch out past logical techniques to issues like informed assent, patient independence, and the dependable direct of clinical preliminaries. Guaranteeing that patients completely comprehend the ramifications of genomic profiling, likely dangers and advantages, and the security concerns related with sharing their hereditary data is

fundamental. Furthermore, addressing differences in admittance to clinical preliminaries and staying away from abuse of weak populaces are principal moral contemplations that require continuous consideration.

The moral components of immunotherapy incorporate contemplations connected with patient determination, informed assent, and the administration of resistant related unfavorable occasions. Choosing proper patients for immunotherapy in view of prescient biomarkers is pivotal for enhancing treatment results. Giving clear and understandable data to patients about the expected advantages and dangers of immunotherapy, particularly given its clever instruments of activity, is fundamental for acquiring informed assent. Overseeing insusceptible related antagonistic occasions morally includes brief acknowledgment, compelling correspondence, and custom fitted intercessions to limit damage to patients.

With regards to fluid biopsy, moral contemplations incorporate issues of informed assent, information possession, and the dependable utilization of hereditary data.

Patients going through fluid biopsy ought to be completely educated about the reasons regarding the test, the likely ramifications of the outcomes, and how their information will be used. Defending patient privacy and forestalling unapproved admittance to hereditary data are basic moral goals. Also, laying out rules for the mindful utilization of fluid biopsy brings about clinical navigation is fundamental to stay away from pointless mediations or unjustifiable uneasiness for patients.

The moral elements of simulated intelligence and AI in malignant growth research include straightforwardness, responsibility, and value. Guaranteeing that simulated intelligence calculations are created and approved utilizing assorted and agent datasets is fundamental to try not to propagate predispositions and variations in medical services. Straightforward detailing of how man-made intelligence models come to explicit end results or expectations is basic for encouraging trust among medical services suppliers and patients. In addition, tending to the potential for work dislodging in fields like pathology, where artificial intelligence driven diagnostics might become common, requires proactive moral contemplations and systems for labor force variation.

In the investigation of the growth microenvironment, moral contemplations spin around acquiring informed assent for research including human subjects, particularly while getting to and concentrating on cancer tissue. Regarding patient independence, guaranteeing protection, and keeping up with classification are fundamental moral standards. Also, while considering helpful intercessions that regulate the growth microenvironment, moral contemplations incorporate limiting damage to typical tissues and offsetting possible advantages with gambles.

The moral difficulties in malignant growth examination and treatment likewise stretch out to the domain of manufactured lethality and designated treatments. Distinguishing and approving manufactured deadly collaborations frequently includes preclinical examinations utilizing cell lines and creature models.

Moral contemplations remember the mindful utilization of creatures for research, guaranteeing altruistic treatment, and making an interpretation of discoveries to clinical preliminaries with fitting moral oversight. Besides, as designated treatments move towards clinical application, issues of patient choice, informed assent, and the impartial conveyance of novel medicines come to the very front of moral contemplations.

Multi-omics mix raises moral contemplations connected with information sharing, cooperation, and the dependable utilization of patient data. As scientists join genomics, transcriptomics, proteomics, and metabolomics information, guaranteeing the protection and security of these multi-layered datasets turns into a principal moral concern. Executing vigorous information administration structures, acquiring informed assent for multi-omics exploration, and cultivating straightforward coordinated effort are fundamental for maintaining moral norms in the period of extensive atomic profiling.

The microbiome's job in disease research acquaints moral contemplations related with microbiome-based mediations. As analysts investigate the capability of balancing the stomach microbiome to improve malignant growth treatment results, moral standards of patient independence, informed assent, and limiting potential dangers become an integral factor. Guaranteeing that patients are completely educated about the objectives, expected advantages, and vulnerabilities of microbiome-based mediations is urgent for maintaining moral guidelines in translational examination.

Metabolic weaknesses as an objective for malignant growth treatment raise moral contemplations as far as potential off-target impacts and long haul results. Balancing explicit metabolic pathways to specifically target disease cells requires cautious thought of the effect on ordinary cells and tissues. Moral standards of limiting damage, acquiring informed assent, and straightforwardly imparting possible dangers and advantages become urgent as metabolic-designated treatments progress from preclinical improvement to clinical preliminaries.

The moral difficulties in engineered lethality research include the dependable utilization of hereditary data and expected ramifications for patients. Recognizing manufactured deadly connections frequently depends on hereditary profiling of cancers, and moral contemplations incorporate acquiring informed assent for genomic investigations and straightforward correspondence of discoveries. As engineered deadly treatments move towards clinical application, guaranteeing impartial access, keeping away from abuse, and consolidating patient viewpoints become fundamental parts of moral navigation.

In the domain of customized disease antibodies, moral contemplations rotate around understanding independence, informed assent, and the dependable lead of clinical preliminaries. Patients going through inoculation ought to be completely educated about the reasoning, expected advantages, and dangers related with customized disease antibodies.

Guaranteeing that the plan and execution of clinical preliminaries stick to moral norms, including evenhanded member choice and thorough oversight, is central for maintaining the standards of examination morals.

As man-made consciousness and AI keep on molding malignant growth research, moral contemplations should advance couple. Issues of straightforwardness, responsibility, and predisposition alleviation become progressively basic as simulated intelligence calculations impact clinical independent direction. Guaranteeing that these innovations are created and conveyed morally requires interdisciplinary joint effort, continuous assessment, and a pledge to maintaining the best expectations of patient consideration and security.

In the investigation of the cancer microenvironment, moral contemplations envelop the dependable direct of examination including human subjects, particularly while acquiring and concentrating on growth tissue tests. Regarding patient independence, acquiring informed assent, and protecting security are primary moral standards. Furthermore, while considering remedial mediations that tweak the growth microenvironment, moral contemplations incorporate limiting mischief to ordinary tissues, offsetting expected benefits with dangers, and directing clinical preliminaries with thorough moral oversight.

The moral difficulties in malignant growth exploration and treatment additionally reach out to the domain of engineered lethality and designated treatments. Distinguishing and approving engineered deadly communications frequently includes preclinical investigations utilizing cell lines and creature models. Moral contemplations remember the mindful utilization of creatures for research, guaranteeing sympathetic treatment, and making an interpretation of discoveries to clinical preliminaries with proper moral oversight. Additionally, as designated treatments move towards clinical application, issues of patient determination, informed assent, and the impartial conveyance of novel medicines come to the very front of moral contemplations.

Multi-omics mix raises moral contemplations connected with information sharing, cooperation, and the capable utilization of patient data. As specialists join genomics, transcriptomics, proteomics, and metabolomics information, guaranteeing the protection and security of these multi-faceted datasets turns into a fundamental moral concern. Carrying out powerful information administration structures, getting educated assent for multi-omics examination, and cultivating straightforward coordinated effort are fundamental for maintaining moral guidelines in the period of complete atomic profiling.

The microbiome's part in disease research acquaints moral contemplations related with microbiome-based mediations. As analysts investigate the capability of adjusting the stomach microbiome to improve malignant growth treatment results, moral standards of patient independence, informed assent, and limiting potential dangers become possibly the most important factor.

Guaranteeing that patients are completely educated about the objectives, expected advantages, and vulnerabilities of microbiome-based mediations is significant for maintaining moral guidelines in translational exploration.

Metabolic weaknesses as an objective for malignant growth treatment raise moral contemplations as far as potential off-target impacts and long haul results. Tweaking explicit metabolic pathways to specifically target malignant growth cells requires cautious thought of the effect on typical cells and tissues. Moral standards of limiting damage, getting educated assent, and straightforwardly conveying expected dangers and advantages become urgent as metabolic-designated treatments progress from preclinical improvement to clinical preliminaries.

The moral difficulties in engineered lethality research include the dependable utilization of hereditary data and expected ramifications for patients. Recognizing manufactured deadly connections frequently depends on hereditary profiling of cancers, and moral contemplations incorporate acquiring informed assent for genomic investigations and straightforward correspondence of discoveries. As engineered deadly treatments move towards clinical application, guaranteeing impartial access, keeping away from abuse, and consolidating patient viewpoints become fundamental parts of moral navigation.

In the domain of customized disease antibodies, moral contemplations rotate around quiet independence, informed assent, and the mindful direct of clinical preliminaries. Patients going through inoculation ought to be completely educated about the reasoning, likely advantages, and dangers related with customized malignant growth immunizations. Guaranteeing that the plan and execution of clinical preliminaries stick to moral guidelines, including evenhanded member determination and thorough oversight, is central for maintaining the standards of examination morals.

As man-made reasoning and AI keep on forming malignant growth research, moral contemplations should develop pair. Issues of straightforwardness, responsibility, and inclination moderation become progressively basic as man-made intelligence calculations impact clinical direction. Guaranteeing that these innovations are created and conveyed morally requires interdisciplinary joint effort, progressing assessment, and a pledge to maintaining the best expectations of patient consideration and protection.

The investigation of the cancer microenvironment, with its perplexing interaction of various cell parts, raises moral contemplations connected with research including human subjects. Getting educated assent for getting to and concentrating on cancer tissue is essential, regarding patient independence and guaranteeing security. Moreover, while creating helpful mediations focusing on the growth microenvironment, moral contemplations incorporate limiting mischief to typical tissues, offsetting expected benefits with dangers, and leading clinical preliminaries with thorough moral oversight.

9.3 Call to action for continued innovation in cancer treatment strategies

The quickly developing scene of malignant growth examination and treatment requests an unflinching source of inspiration to cultivate proceeded with development. While amazing steps have been made in understanding the sub-atomic complexities of malignant growth and creating designated treatments, the complicated and heterogeneous nature of the illness requires progressing endeavors to push the limits of logical revelation and clinical practice. This source of inspiration reaches out across different spaces, incorporating research, innovation, joint effort, and a guarantee to tending to the different difficulties that lie ahead.

At the very front of the source of inspiration is the basic for supported interest in disease research. Powerful subsidizing is the backbone of logical request, empowering scientists to investigate novel speculations, lead thorough analyses, and make an interpretation of disclosures into substantial clinical headways. Government offices, generous associations, and confidential area elements should keep on assigning assets to help fundamental and translational examination that unwinds the secrets of malignant growth science and recognizes imaginative restorative targets.

The source of inspiration likewise highlights the requirement for a cooperative and interdisciplinary way to deal with malignant growth research. Separating storehouses and encouraging cooperation among analysts, clinicians, computational scholars, and information researchers is fundamental for handling the complex difficulties presented by malignant growth. Cooperative drives that unite specialists from assorted fields work with the incorporation of genomic information, clinical bits of knowledge, and mechanical developments, making ready for comprehensive ways to deal with malignant growth determination and treatment.

Mechanical development is a key part in the source of inspiration for propelling malignant growth treatment systems. Proceeded with interest in state of the art advancements, for example, man-made reasoning, AI, and high-throughput genomics is basic. These innovations not just improve our capacity to investigate immense datasets yet in addition empower the distinguishing proof of unpretentious examples and affiliations that might evade customary scientific methodologies. Coordinating these innovative advances into clinical practice holds the commitment of more exact diagnostics, customized treatment designs, and worked on tolerant results.

The source of inspiration reaches out to the domain of accuracy medication, stressing the significance of fitting disease medicines in light of the one of a kind hereditary cosmetics of every patient's growth. Genomic profiling and sub-atomic portrayal enable oncologists to choose designated treatments that explicitly address the hereditary modifications driving a singular's disease.

This customized approach has proactively shown outcome in specific disease types, and the source of inspiration includes growing these endeavors to cover a more extensive range of malignancies, guaranteeing that more patients can profit from accuracy oncology.

Immunotherapy, proclaimed as an extraordinary methodology in malignant growth treatment, requests a reverberating source of inspiration for additional innovative work. While immunotherapy has shown striking adequacy in certain patients, difficulties, for example, treatment opposition and resistant related antagonistic occasions continue. The source of inspiration includes unwinding the intricacies of the growth microenvironment, grasping the systems of opposition, and creating procedures to upgrade the strength of immunotherapy reactions. Furthermore, growing the utilization of immunotherapy to at present less responsive malignant growth types stays a basic objective.

Fluid biopsy, as a painless indicative instrument, calls for proceeded with development to upgrade its responsiveness, particularity, and clinical utility. The source of inspiration includes refining fluid biopsy methods to recognize negligible lingering sickness, screen therapy reactions progressively, and illuminate remedial direction. Normalization of fluid biopsy strategies and the foundation of clear rules for result understanding are fundamental to successfully incorporate this creative methodology into routine clinical practice.

Man-made reasoning (artificial intelligence) and AI, as vital parts of the source of inspiration, hold huge potential in changing malignant growth analysis and treatment.

The improvement of simulated intelligence calculations equipped for dissecting assorted datasets, including genomics, clinical imaging, and clinical records, is urgent. The source of inspiration underscores the significance of thorough approval, straightforwardness, and moral contemplations in the organization of man-made intelligence driven advances to guarantee their mindful reconciliation into clinical work processes.

The source of inspiration stretches out to tending to variations in disease care and guaranteeing fair admittance to creative medicines. Endeavors to overcome any issues in medical services abberations include executing strategies that focus on inclusivity, eliminating obstructions to get to, and advancing variety in clinical preliminaries. Furthermore, the source of inspiration incorporates the improvement of techniques to make progressed disease therapies more reasonable and open all around the world, lessening the weight of malignant growth on patients and medical services frameworks.

In the investigation of the microbiome's part in malignant growth, the source of inspiration includes disentangling the perplexing connections between the stomach microbiome and disease advancement. Understanding how the microbiome impacts reactions to malignant growth treatments and investigating intercessions to regulate the microbiome for helpful advantage are fundamental parts of this source of inspiration.

Continuous examination in this space holds the possibility to open new roads for further developing therapy results and tending to the difficulties presented by the microbiome-disease pivot.

Metabolic weaknesses as focuses for disease treatment highlight the source of inspiration for inventive procedures that specifically target malignant growth cell digestion. Growing little particles or other remedial modalities that upset explicit metabolic pathways in disease cells while saving typical cells is a key concentration. The source of inspiration likewise includes making an interpretation of preclinical discoveries into clinical preliminaries to assess the wellbeing and adequacy of metabolic-designated treatments in different malignant growth types.

Manufactured lethality, as a promising road for designated malignant growth treatments, requests a source of inspiration for additional investigation of hereditary collaborations and the improvement of novel restorative procedures. Recognizing manufactured deadly collaborations, approving them in preclinical models, and making an interpretation of these discoveries into clinical applications comprise the center of this source of inspiration. The objective is to extend the collection of accuracy treatments that exploit the extraordinary hereditary weaknesses of disease cells.

The source of inspiration envelops a guarantee to tending to moral contemplations in malignant growth examination and treatment. Guaranteeing informed assent, safeguarding patient security, and cultivating straightforwardness in the utilization of genomic and clinical information are essential moral objectives. The source of inspiration reaches out to advancing inclusivity and variety in research, clinical preliminaries, and the improvement of creative treatments, mirroring a pledge to moral rules that focus on value and equity in disease care.

Instruction and mindfulness structure an essential piece of the source of inspiration. Enabling medical care experts, scientists, and the overall population with modern information about arising patterns in disease research cultivates a cooperative and informed approach. The source of inspiration includes putting resources into instructive projects, public effort drives, and gatherings that work with information trade, empowering a common perspective of the difficulties and potential open doors in the field of malignant growth exploration and treatment.

www.ingramcontent.com/pod-product-compliance
Lightning Source LLC
Chambersburg PA
CBHW071649210326
41597CB00017B/2161

* 9 7 8 0 7 1 9 9 8 7 3 8 0 *